Sleazy Stories III

Sleazy Stories III

A Seducer's Stream of Thots

Aaron Sleazy

Black Swallowtail Publishing

© Aaron Sleazy 2019
http://www.aaronsleazy.com

Proofreading by A.S.Y. and Chris Griffith.

Revision 1.00

ISBN 978-3-942017-07-7

To all you horny men, again

Contents

Preface

It is quite surprising how good you can get at something if you fully devote yourself to it. Not bothering with holding down a real job, I spent most of my time in 2009 chasing after women. While the average Joe may be able to go out once every other week I was out and about several times a week. Looking back I still find it staggering how much of an infrastructure for people not spending eight hours a day in an office building Berlin provides. If you wanted to, you could go out and get laid basically every single day of the week. Monday would have provided a veritable challenge but on any other night you were spoiled for choice.

Going out and getting laid is one thing; the nine-to-five grind is already incompatible with partying until 4:00 a.m., taking some girl home and, after plenty of fun and a few hours of sleep, finally getting up sometime in the afternoon. There is also the fact that there are a lot of women who need a lover with a flexible schedule to get their sexual needs met. That was me back in the days, putting my libido above everything else.

Sleazy Stories III continues a few days after the end of *Sleazy Stories II* and covers most of my hook-ups from just one month, mid-May to mid-June 2009. You may think that there is not so much that can happen in one month but I can assure you there is: nymphomaniacs, sluts who cheat on their boyfriend or husband, empowered women who believe they can tell me what to do and how to act, an insecure woman who thinks that all she can offer is sex, masterful cocksuckers, incompetent cocksuckers, a lingerie model with borderline personality disorder, a good Christian girl, a submissive Asian cutie, and more await you in these pages. This book is a wild romp and I hope you will enjoy it even more than the previous ones.

AARON SLEAZY

Orgasm Girl

I am not quite sure why I keep picking up girls with the goal of banging them in bathroom stalls, on parking lots or behind dumpsters. I am no longer after just sex. Don't get me wrong: I like sex. In fact, I am probably a sex addict. However, calling one of my fuck buddies and telling her to come over is just so different from going out, meeting some woman, and fucking her before the break of dawn.

After my encounter with a girl I referred to as one of the biggest sluts of Berlin — you can read about her in the last chapter of *Sleazy Stories II* — I got some self-doubts. I certainly do not mind the attention I get from all those sluts, but reflecting on the morals of those women readily cheating on their boyfriend or husband fills me with disgust. It is quite sobering to look into the abyss modern Western women open up for you. (You can take that literally if you want.) It is another to know that you are one of the beneficiaries of them having loose morals. Well, I keep telling myself that if I do not fuck them then somebody else will. That is not necessarily true, but that is how I like to view it.

After taking it easy for a few days I told my two fuck buddies to come over on Wednesday. No, not at the same time. One at 7 p.m., the other at 11 p.m. The first one I had to kick out after two hours. She was starting to feel a bit too comfortable. I do not mind her company. I rather much enjoy it, in fact, but I had the other chick come over soon. Here is a pro tip: Of course we guys cannot fuck all the time. We need some time off to recharge. However, fucking two different women soon after another is a lot easier than fucking the same old chick one more time. I am getting carried away again. Anyway, on Wednesday I banged my two chicks. On Thursday I wanted some variety again.

Thursday started great. I get up at 8 a.m., tell my chick to give me a morning blow job, and send her off. Then I called in sick at work and went back to bed. At noon I get up for real, treating myself to a proper breakfast before relaxing in the living room, reading romantic poetry. No, seriously! When I wanted to fix myself something to eat for dinner my flatmate NUMBERS came home. We cooked and ate together.

NUMBERS is in a strangely confident mood, almost an exuberant one, so he challenges me to a game of chess.

The cheek! I am not a particularly good player, but if you have never seriously studied the game I will wipe the floor with you. That was also the fate he was about to face yet again. Somehow he thinks that it is due to bad luck when he loses. Instead, I am still cashing in dividends from a book on pawn structures in chess I worked through years ago. It is written by a guy called Kmoch, if I recall correctly. I should teach my flatmate a thing or two about that topic. Then again, when I offered to lend him my copy of Tarrasch's *The Game of Chess* he was not interested. After my victory on the chess board I take a well-deserved nap.

I wake up at around 11:30 p.m. with some kind of late-evening boner. That is motivation enough for me to go out and get laid. So here we go again. I make it to the station just in time to hop on the last tram departing from my corner in Prenzlauer Berg for the day. This allows me to travel conveniently to Sage Club in Kreuzberg. You know that place. We have been there together already. I am glad that I manage to get there. Otherwise, I would have been forced to drop by one of the smaller clubs closer to my place, such as Magnet Club. It is not a bad venue, but there is just not the same quantity of women. Quality-wise they are pretty comparable, so that is not an issue. But quantity is, as the crowd at Sage Club is many times bigger. I arrive at Sage Club at around 1:00 a.m. The queue is enormous as it is often the case if you show up around that time.

After half an hour I am finally inside.

Sage Club is massive. On Thursdays they host a few bands but of course no big acts. This normally draws quite a crowd. Also, they let you in for free if you show up before 10:00 p.m., or is it 9:00 p.m.? I don't know. That is way too early anyway. There are three dance floors, which they gradually open, but it is not a fun venue if it is not packed. You can get unlucky even if you show up at a saner time, like me. Tonight they are playing indie rock on the main floor, hard rock on the second one, and on the small one downstairs some DJ with a predilection for the relative cutting edge in popular music has been trying his luck. At least that is what I think. I do not follow the scene that much anymore, compared to my time in London.

I am having a great time downstairs. The music is fun. The moment I start to dance some girl turns around and mirrors my movements. Her boyfriend does not like that and drags her off while she keeps staring at me. Compared to her boyfriend I think I am the better choice in every conceivable way, minus the money part maybe. Heck, in Berlin about a quarter of the working-age population is living off welfare and I do not even qualify for that. Thus, I am competitive on that front as well, even though I am a fucking loser.

I head upstairs and walk past a row of sofas. A cute girl gives me a warm smile, so I sit down next to her right away and throw an arm around her. She laughs and cuddles up to me before putting a bit of distance between us. You know, they cannot make it too easy for you! I do not really remember what we were talking about but she has a really bubbly personality and I like her. She has a pendant between her perky breasts that is shaped like a cat. I take it into my grubby hand to have a closer look at it but as I lean forward I somehow end up pressing the back of my hand against one of her breasts and rub it. We make deep eye contact.

"Why does your cat have a leg shaped like a cock?", I ask her.

"Like a what?", she retorts incredulously, before laughing hysterically.

"If you just squint a little bit the paw totally looks like the tip of a cock."

She keeps laughing.

"That's not all! The whiskers look like pubic hair so your cat basically has a dick growing out of her face."

She is in stitches and then she playfully slaps my chest.

"Did you make this?", I ask her.

"Who, me? I couldn't do that. I got it at Oxfam a couple of years ago."

"I guess it's good you're not designing jewelry. It would be cocks around the clock otherwise."

(I was really proud of that pun as jewelry makers may try their hand at designing clocks or pocket watches, but I am afraid that my sophisticated humor flew right past her.)

"You didn't just say that, did you?", she says and keeps laughing as she is caressing my chest.

"Sure did," I say with a serious look on my face.

"You're great! But let me get some fresh air. I'll be right back. Please wait for me here."

I do not feel like jeopardizing this interaction. She is pretty horny and who knows whom else she might run into.

"Now that you mention it I could use some fresh air, too."

I take her hand and lead her to the outdoor area. She is squeezing my hand. I would say she is pretty into me. I do not like the outdoor area much, though. It is cold, and some people are smoking. We chit-chat for a bit. Now a male friend of hers joins us, presumably some orbiter. This kills the mood. He overheard that we were talking about music, which is his excuse to drone on and on about some band none of us has ever heard of.

My phone vibrates. It is my Norwegian buddy and seducer extraordinaire TEEVSTER! His family is well-off and gives him free rein, so I am not sure whether he is still in Berlin or whether he just flew in for a long weekend. He dropped me a vague text message earlier this week about going out together, but neither of us is great at making precise plans days in advance. I am happy to hear from him, so I take his call. It is too loud. I cannot understand a single word he says. I tell that woman that I have to take this call and that I will be right back. I am looking for a quiet corner, which is no easy feat but I manage. Now I am in the hallway leading to the main dance floor. I chat with TEEVSTER, telling him where I am and that I would be very happy if he came by. Otherwise I will see him tomorrow or so, or whenever he is back in Berlin.

I put my phone down. As I look up I notice a really cute girl with long black hair smiling at me. I smile back. I do not get to say anything because she blurts out, "Do you want one of my glow sticks?" Before I can say anything she takes one glow stick off her arm and puts it on my wrist. We banter for a bit. Then the girl standing next to her whom I had paid no attention to at all walks off abruptly.

"That's my girlfriend. I think she is jealous."

"She didn't happen to lose some kind of bet, did she?"

She laughs and adds, "I thought guys don't know about such things!"

"So the answer is yes?"

She laughs.

"How about we dance?", I suggest. Before she can say anything I am already leading her downstairs to the dark little dance floor. We are getting quite close, at least physically. While she seems to really enjoy rubbing her pussy against my leg, she turns her head when I try to kiss her. I am surprised by her alleged shyness but just keep at it. I think I could get her number, meet her for coffee, and take it from there, but that is too time-consuming. Thus, I have to see how far I can get right here, right now. I sense that she is getting a bit too uncomfortable. Moments later she excuses herself.

"I really have to get back to my friend!"

She does not seem to dislike me for my boldness. In fact, she hugs me and covers my cheeks with kisses.

"No worries. We can dance some more later," she says.

"Yeah, we should!"

She kisses me again on the cheek, close to my mouth, but my lips are apparently off-limits for her. Anyway, I do not have any intention of continuing with her later but she is fun and I am happy to have made her night.

I turn around and see a really hot chick dancing in a very seductive way. If she wants attention, she can get it. I pull her in and she uses me as some kind of prop for her dance routine. Her hands are all over my body. I am likewise exploring her tight body. Her skin feels great. But now the song is over. She scuttles off to some guy standing at the periphery of the dance floor.

Not all my interactions go great. Plenty do because I have a great eye for spotting girls who are into me. Sometimes, though, I take a risk. It also happens that male and female friends of theirs intervene, or romantic partners. This is what happened later: I am just having fun, spinning a few random girls around, playfully poking two or three in the side, just to provoke a hopefully positive reaction. That is not smooth, but it sometimes does the trick. A girl with huge knockers smiles at me. I take this as the invitation it is and walk up to her. Sadly, she is pretty average overall. Her tits are massive, but her face is plain and her thighs are a bit too thick. That being said, we are talking about a woman with a genuinely voluptuous body, not some chick who is just fat and believes that to be the same as being curvy. It does not take long until her friends start panicking and shield her from me. Young girls and their constant chaperoning each other!

Let me do some very crude foreshadowing and introduce a girl with the telling name ORGASMS. I spot her in the crowd and feel drawn to her. I playfully poke her tummy to check whether she really is in shape. This makes her protest playfully. I shrug and walk off. A little while later I return and take her hand as I walk past, followed by a spin. I keep holding her hand and try walking off with her. She is not having any of it and pulls her hand back. This does not happen in any kind of hostile way, mind you. I make a mental note to maybe continue with her later. After all, I am after a stronger initial reaction.

I am still looking for a girl who is into me right off the bat. There is a group of five girls dancing in a circle. I walk right into it. One of them makes piercing eye contact with me, so that is the one I am focussing on. She is young, cute, and skinny just like all her friends, which means that it does not really matter which one I pick. I take her hand and pull her in. She plunges forward and softens the impact of jumping into me with her breasts. She is really light. I easily lift her up with one arm. She wraps her legs around me.

"Actually, I really don't like any of this," she claimed.

"Yeah, I can tell."

She giggles.

We just stare into each other's eyes. Her friends seem to not matter to her for a moment or two. Then she returns to the real world.

"Okay, that was fun. Now please let me down."

"It's not as if I'm forcing you."

I only have a hand on her ass to support her, of course.

She giggles, "Of course not."

Now she is standing right next to me.

"Um, I'm actually not allowed to do any of this since I have a boyfriend."

I ignore that and drag her off the dance floor. My intention is to get her to a sofa and take this interaction further. She is cute, very slender and in shape. I bet her naked body looks amazing.

"Where are you taking me?"

I keep mum. She keeps walking with me. We are in front of a sofa.

"Sit down!", I say as I put my arm around her and gently guide her.

"I really shouldn't be doing this. I don't think I should sit down with you."

"Come on, it's just for a bit."

I have an arm around her waist. I feel her hand on my neck.

"I'd rather dance some more."

We do not sit down and instead head back to the dance floor. I would not say that we are dancing. She does little more than press her body tightly against mine, and I get to smell her lovely skin. Her hair smells great, too. I have no idea where her friends are and neither does she, but she does not seem to care. She is quite something looks-wise, so I decide to keep working on her.

My new goal is to wear her down gradually. I almost would have said, "tear her down." Yup, I am certainly imagining myself ravaging her already.

I grab her ass and squeeze it. She calmly clenches my wrist and indicates that I should move my hand further up. She is indeed a bit tense, so I transition from her firm ass to her lower back, which she is much more appreciative of. Grabbing her ass like a caveman is a no-no, but she is having no issue at all rubbing her pussy against my thigh. She is also fine with my fingertips tracing her body, including her small and firm breasts. She is getting really into it.

"You're quite a charmer," she says.

"I take this as a compliment."

"I have no idea how you manage to make me do this with you."

(Practice.)

I do not say anything. Instead, we caress each other.

"I think you're way too forward," she says gently and softly.

"Just enjoy it. I know you're not getting much of this."

She looks at me, unsure of what to say.

"You know that I'm right," I add.

She nods and looks down to the floor.

I hear her whisper, "How do you ...?"

"Shh!"

I take her hand and lead her into another room. We sit down on a sofa. She first sits down next to me, but then I lift her up and put her into my lap.

"I really have a boyfriend. I'm not making this up."

I nod.

She gently traces my chest with her index and middle finger.

"I ... , I'm not allowed to do any of this. I'm really not."

She is a tough nut to crack. I lean forward to kiss her neck. She puts her hand on my cheek and pushes me away, but not at all convincingly.

"No!", she whispers.

"Just relax and enjoy it."

She does not say anything but instead closes her eyes. I kiss her neck gently and work my way up to her earlobe. She is melting. I suck on her earlobe, then I lick her ear. I feel her hands on the skin of my back. Then I suck her neck. This prompts her to bury her nails in my back. We look into each other's eyes. Then she comes back to her senses and gets up.

"I really, really ... . No, don't get me wrong. I think you're great. You're amazing. I'd love to ... . I mean, if

I didn't have a boyfriend, I ..., I'm not making this up. I really do have a boyfriend."

She seems a bit confused. I get up as well and embrace her. She wraps her arms around me.

"If I don't leave now, I don't know what will happen," she philosophizes.

I gently kiss her lips. She initially reciprocates, but then forces herself to stop.

"I shouldn't. I ... , I really need to go. Please let me go."

She is turning cold now. I can sense her body stiffening. Consequently, I stop embracing her.

"Not tonight, I mean ... . I have to get back to my friends. "

She looks at me expectantly. I think this is my cue to ask her for her contact details but I do not want to bother with dates if there is not a very high probability that I will get laid with little effort.

"Okay. Have fun," I say.

"You too. You were great!"

"You too!"

She turns around and hurries back to her girlfriends.

I sit down on the sofa for a little bit and just relax. After a while I get up and wander around the venue. The shitty indie bands have long stopped playing and now people are dancing on the stage. That is normally not allowed. Yet, too many people — read: cute women — are doing it to make security stop them. One security guy stands right next to the stage, making sure that nobody accidentally falls off.

That girl I had run into earlier, ORGASMS, is also dancing on the stage. Some guy is trying to get her attention by awkwardly dancing about three feet away from her, and not directly facing her either. What a loser! I walk straight up to her and pull her in. Her hands are instantly all over me. She has been waiting for someone to hit on her. Probably more or less anyone would have sufficed, given how horny she is. ORGASMS is pressing her tits against my body. From the corner of my eye I see the other dude walking off with his tail between his legs.

I am teasing her a bit by leaning in for a kiss. Because she immediately goes for it I pull my head back and grin mischievously. She gives me a really horny look in return. She is not wearing a bra, so her tube top is doing a poor job of trying to hide her stiff nipples. I tickle one of them and laugh. That is enough playing around for now, though. To reward her for how she has been looking at me, I grab her by the neck, pull her in, and tongue her down hard. We are about one to two minutes in, for your information.

We are making out. Her hands are under my T-shirt,

squeezing and scratching my back. I roll her tube top up a little bit and lift my T-shirt up, before pressing our exposed sweaty midriffs together. (Some horny slut in London taught me that move. Moments later she had one hand in my pants and was stroking my cock.) We are still making out. I pull back so that I do not give her too much of a sexual release. She grabs my hair with one hand and tries pulling my head down to her. I am a tall guy. She is about ten inches shorter than me and that is in her heels, so that is not going to work out. She instinctively gets on her toes, which looks comical as she is not gaining much, given the kind of shoes she is wearing.

She still has one hand on the back of my head and she is excessively eager to kiss me. I lean in and pull back right afterward — only to grab her mane and pull her head back. I lick her neck. She moans. I go for the kiss. As soon as she opens her mouth I shove my tongue down her throat. Then I playfully push her away while making strong eye contact. Of course, she is coming right back to me. We stare into each other's eyes. She is so horny that I could just bend her over and fuck her if we were not on the stage, exposing ourselves to a few hundred people dancing around us. Then I notice a curtain in the corner of the stage. I have no idea what is behind it. It is time to find out.

I take her hand, quickly walk toward the curtain with

her, and peek behind it. It is a storage room, which is a great place to continue my interaction with that little slut. There are some big crates piled up. I notice several monitors, an amp, and a few instruments. All of this stuff must belong to tonight's bands. There is an adjacent room, too. I see people walking back and forth, carrying stuff. Those might be roadies or maybe they are band members doing the job of roadies. Well, they can do their thing. I will do mine. I lead her over to a wall. The view is partly blocked by two crates that are stacked on top of each other. My head is sticking out behind those crates but she will be invisible once she squats down.

I presume she is thinking what I am thinking. I lean against the wall. She grabs my head with both hands and tongues me down hard. Meanwhile, I grab her by the pussy and rub her crotch passionately. Putting one and one together, I realize that I may as well just pull my cock out. We are making out passionately. She has both hands in my hair. I have one hand on her crotch. With the other I unbutton and then unzip my pants. I take one of her hands and put it onto my cock, which is pretty hard already. She is whacking me while we are making out. This is not really doing it for me for long, so I pull my boxers and pants down a little bit, put one hand on the top of her head and push her down. She gets the hint right away and is downright plunging down on my cock with her mouth open. Her first move is a deep throat!

She has just been waiting for me to let her suck my dick. Now we are about five minutes in. I am setting new personal bests here. I shove one of my hands into her tube top and briefly wonder if I will end up wrecking it. I squeeze one of her marvelous breasts with my left hand, with the other I have a tight hold of her mane and yank her head back and forth, frequently shoving it all the way down so that she can impress me with her deep-throating skills. She makes gargling sounds. When I yank her back she gasps for air, only to get my massive stiff cock down her throat once again. All I have heard from her thus far are moans and "Mmmm." I do not enjoy talking with women as I tend to find them to be shallow conversationalist, but what this girl has been uttering is the kind of communication with women I do not seem to ever get tired of.

I let her feast on my massive boner some more. I am hitting the back of her throat with the tip of my cock and feel her tongue working on my shaft at the same time. She is making deep eye contact. Cute chicks with my dick in their mouth looking at me lustfully is something I thoroughly appreciate. Bitch all you want about women's liberation, but the fact of the matter is that I am getting sex for free with ease. My father's generation, maybe my grandfather's generation, had to pay for hookers. Today sluts fuck you for validation, which is pretty crazy if you think about it, considering that after blowing a load you could not care less about such a chick.

It is cramped in that storage room and leaning against the wall is not particularly comfortable, but I let her continue. I have a hunch that she is good enough at sucking dick to make me come with her mouth alone. I should probably find a more comfortable position. Sitting down somewhere would be good. Right now there is not much space. We are pretty squeezed in. Well, time to rearrange ourselves. As I am still grabbing her by the hair on the back of her head, I just yank her head back. She looks at my erect penis. For good measure I take my dick and slap her in the face with it. The second time I want to do it she tries to evade it and in turn takes it into her mouth again. That is enough of an intermission. I stretch her out, a bit like an accordion, by pulling her head upward. We make deep eye contact. I move her sideways, where there is a bit more space. Before I can say anything she grabs my balls with one hand and my neck with the other and shoves her tongue down my throat. Now she has one hand on my dick. With the other she is playing with my balls.

I gesture her to squat down again by putting one hand on her head and pushing her down. She is now squatting and presumably readying herself for the grand finale. Then a roadie walks by and shouts, "Hey, you're not supposed to be in here. Get the fuck out!"

Because she was squatting down he has seen only me. That must have been an odd sight, seeing a dude's head sticking out in a messy storage area.

"Sorry, mate!", I say in return.

As I look down again I notice that my chick is gone. She could not keep her cool. The curtain that blocks the view to the stage is moving. Man, I had such a nice hard-on! Anyway, I pack it away, fix my clothes and head back on stage, looking for ORGASMS. She is on the other side of the curtain, trying to act as if nothing had happened. As soon as she sees me we are making out again. It is really time I get this over and done with, so I take her hand and lead her — yes, exactly! — to the bathroom stalls.

We are in the men's restroom. All the stalls are occupied. There is a urinal next to the stalls and guys are walking back and forth. It is not the most romantic environment you could think of, that is for sure. In order to combat the dreary reality of this pickup I make out with her. After a moment or two she gently pushes me back. At first I do not know what this is about, but then it is clear. She picked up that someone was about to leave the bathroom stall as she has heard the unlocking movement of the lever before opening the door. I am really impressed! I did not pick up on that. Then again, I had focused on the big picture, i.e., door movement.

Some dude walks out. I keep the door open and usher her in. Then I walk in and lock the door behind me. As I turn around she throws her arms around me and tongues me down hard. She grabs my hair and pulls it. With the other hand she scratches my back. I unbuckle my belt and pull my pants down. She is very perceptive and does not need further instructions. She sits down on the toilet seat, grabs my ass cheeks, and gets to work. Glory times!

She is not doing her racy deep-throats so much. Instead, she is sucking my dick slowly and methodologically. Once I am really hard she is speeding up. I liked her really slutty side better, so I grab her by the hair on the back of her head, pull her head back and slap her in the face with my hard cock. One. Two. Three. Four. Five. Then I lift her up and shove her against the wall, mid-air. She is moaning. I let her down. With one hand I am choking her, with the other I am in her pants, fingering her. It is surreal how incredibly turned on she is getting. Her face is red. She also has a flush on her chest and she is so wet that I have to wipe my fingers on her top in between because it is getting too slippery. I do not think I have ever seen a reaction like that from a woman I am dominating. By now we still have not exchanged a single word. Now I notice that it seems there is menstrual blood on my fingers. I keep going nonetheless.

She rolls up her tube top to expose her ripe breasts. I suck on her nipples while I am pressing her against the wall. My right forearm is against her neck, my left hand is grabbing and massaging her pussy. Her moaning is getting out of control. Thankfully we are in a loud nightclub. I am hitting her G-spot, then I am pulling my fingers out of her dripping pussy to give her some room to breathe. She is panting. I gesture her to sit down, before grabbing her head and shoving it onto my cock again.

I am getting my dick sucked pretty well. She really knows how to do it. Yet, even after a few minutes she still has not managed to make me come just with her mouth. Thus, I pull her head back and yank my dick out of her mouth. I am whacking myself while she lustfully stares at my big dick. I am getting close to blowing a load. As I am close to the point of no return I shove my dick into her mouth again. Now I need very little extra effort to get over the edge and we are about to get there. She is sucking the tip of my cock, tugging my balls with one hand, and whacking my cock with the other. We are done! I am coming. As I am shooting my wad down her throat she utters some muffled "Mmmmm"-sounds. A big load is now making its way through her body. I am feeling great. I smile but not necessarily at her. I just smile and pant.

She is looking up at me. On her face is an expression of utter bliss. It is just beautiful to look at her. This looks like a clear win-win to me. Then again, maybe my perception is off because I have just blown a load. It is not that I care that much anyway. She has now been smiling with a big wide smile at me for what felt like around a minute or two. Finally, she laughs and says, "Oh my God!" I smile some more. We are making out again.

I still have not said anything to her and I am wondering how far my non-verbal communication skills can take me. As a reward for excellent performance I want to do something for her too, so I pull her pants down. (She is still sitting.) She is leaning back. I put my index finger on her lower lip then gently shove it into her mouth, then I put it in as deeply as I can. She is moaning and sucking on it. I pull my index finger out of her mouth and move on to, with the wet tip of it, massaging her clitoris. As she is getting into it I use my other hand to pull the little hat over her clit up in order to properly expose it. I gently and quickly massage it. She starts to moan. It is not just that. She is getting louder and louder. Within about two minutes she is close to coming and still getting louder. Now she is coming and screaming down the entire place. She is like an animal. That is probably not the first time she has a reaction like this because with one hand she grabs my wrist and pulls my hand toward her face. I am about to cover her mouth with my hand, but that is not what she had in mind. Instead, she stuffs all fingers of my hand into her mouth, which muffles her orgasmic screams. At the height of her orgasm her body jerks involuntarily. This is all exceedingly hot. I am getting hard just thinking about it again.

She is panting. I take her into my arms and we embrace each other, melting into one. At this point I will probably lose some of you because you think I am bullshitting. However, what I just told you we repeated a few more times in different variations. We spent well over an hour in total in that dingy bathroom stall. I gave her seven or eight orgasms and I am talking about distinct orgasms, not a couple of multiple ones blending together in one big orgasmic wave. I allowed her to cool down before starting over. I really enjoyed seeing her orgasm, which kept my motivation up.

Let us make the other orgasms a bit quicker. The second one is an accident: She sits down. I want to eventually hammer her G-spot hard, but as I am working toward that I notice that she reacts extremely well to me just playing with her labia, tugging them a bit, caressing them. Out of the blue this snowballs into an orgasm. She could not quite believe that either. For the third one I worked on her clitoris again as I wanted to give her another one and was quite certain that she could reach it this way. It seems she has gotten into a state in which she needed only very little stimulation to come, which I have a hard time wrapping my head around. The fourth one was quite experimental: we are embracing each other tightly. I pull her pants down a little bit and massage a particular part of her ass, somewhere around the 10 o'clock position on the left and the 2 o'clock position on the right. Some women get turned on if you massage that spot. She does not just get turned on. She gets really into it — and collapses, wrapping her arms around me. I am grabbing her to prevent her from falling to the floor. As she is hanging on to me, she orgasms and pants.

I have begun counting her orgasms and feel like the man. It is all strangely satisfying, which surprises me a little bit because I do not think I care that much about the female orgasm. In that regard, she is pretty special. For orgasm no. 5 I want to hammer her G-spot. To make it a bit easier for me I pull her pants down to about her knees. Then I notice a thread coming out of her pussy.

"Could you please remove your tampon?", I ask and that is the first thing I say to her! As I realize this I suppress a chuckle.

"Yeah, sure. Hold on!"

She pulls a blood-soaked tampon out of her pussy and drops it into the toilet bowl. As she is turning around she asks, "Are you sure you want to do this without protection?"

Now that is a statement! She basically invited me to fuck her raw. Plenty of women let you fuck them raw but normally it is nothing they verbalize. Instead, they may pull the condom off your cock or surprise you by quickly sitting down on your cock while you think that foreplay is still going on. One moment she is rubbing her labia over your shaft, the next she is holding the base of your cock and sits down on it, believing that once you feel the sensation of her wet, warm pussy, you will not insist on using a condom anymore.

I have some condoms in my back pocket, but fucking a chick on her period, with or without a condom, is messy. I have no idea how badly she is bleeding and I really do not want to think about the kind of mess I might create. Besides, bloodstains ruin your clothes and traveling home on public transport with bloodstains all over my pants is not something I am keen on ever doing.

"Let me finger you."

"Do you really want to do this, with my period and all that?"

"This turns me on even more."

This is not quite true. Instead, the important point is to keep the momentum going. Imagine a woman offers you her pussy and then you say you do not want to fuck her, followed by saying that you do not want to finger her either. It is a good compromise to get some blood on your hands.

She responds with another one of her beaming smiles, which I find incredibly attractive. I turn her around and slide my fingers in deep. As she is getting very aroused very quickly I curl my index and middle finger and hammer her G-spot, followed by stretching my fingers and sliding them in deep. I hit her G-spot three times, followed by going in all the way one time. Doing this in a consistent rhythm is working quite well. Indeed, moments later she is coming again. By that time I had learned to shove my hand into her mouth before she begins with her orgasmic screams.

She notices that my cock is coming back to life. I am thinking what she is thinking.

"Sit down and lick my balls!", I tell her.

She sits down and gives me a more than decent teabagging while whacking my dick. Then she opens her mouth and slowly slides my dick in all the way. She stares into my eyes but does not move her head. Now she winks — and digs her nails into my ass while deepthroating me like a pro. She does not hold back anything. I am dripping in sweat and so is she. Our reptile brains have taken over.

Unfortunately, she can't quite figure out how to work my dick. She is very good, that is for sure, but this is not the time to teach her what she should do to suck me really well. Now that she has been working hard on sucking my dick I gesture her to stop. Then I whack myself again. I want to shoot another load into her mouth. She gets the hint and immediately squats down in front of me, with her tongue pressing against the tip of my cock. As soon as pre-cum is coming out she wraps her lips around the tip of my cock and sucks really hard on it. It is so hot! I eventually have to stop her because she just keeps sucking, even well after I am done blowing a load. After a while the tip of your cock just gets too sensitive.

She keeps my dick in her mouth, lips wrapped around the tip, but no longer sucks it. Then she takes it out of her mouth, smiles, and swallows my cum. Now she pulls the foreskin of my cock all the way back and holds on to the shaft. She is cleaning my dick properly with her tongue and the cum she picks up that way she swallows as well. Then she looks at me and smiles. After giggling briefly she says again, "Oh. My. God!", but this time with long pauses between the words. She laughs. I help her get up. We hug and caress each other for a while. We are still not talking to each other. We only utter sounds of pleasure.

I am regaining my strength, so I expose her tits again and slowly but gently suck on her nipples, which are really stiff. To my bewilderment, after something like two or three minutes she has an orgasm from that as well. I think I am interacting with some kind of orgasm machine. I was not even aware that women can come from stimulating their nipples. As I later learned, involuntary orgasms are not that uncommon. A few years later a girl in my yoga class had one and got pretty embarrassed by it.

I may even have forgotten one of her orgasms. We were at least at seven. Maybe there was another one that has slipped my mind. After some comforting and caressing I am wondering if I can come again. Glazing her face with a load of cum would be a nice finish, so I pull my dick out and whack it. I am clearly at my limit now, though. She just stares at it with big eyes and her mouth agape. I am not even touching her. She leans against the wall, still panting softly. As I am getting a chubby her eyes are getting even bigger. Then she involuntarily jerks her body, wraps her arms around me and moans loudly.

After she is done with it I ask her, "What was that? Did you just come again?"

"I guess so. It totally felt like it."

Her reaction completely baffled me. (Through subsequent research I learned that this is called a psychological orgasm. They are supposedly pretty rare.)

I did not have enough energy in me to come yet again, so I hug her.

"How often did you come in total? I lost track along the way," I ask.

"I don't know. It's been all a blur to me. Let me think!"

She is closing her eyes and counting with her fingers, which looks pretty cute.

"Mm, I think nine times."

"Is this normal for you?"

She slaps me playfully.

"No, it's not. I have no idea what you have been doing to me. I've never, ever experienced anything like that, like not at all."

After a pause she says, "Can you just hold me?"

She sinks into my arms. She is completely worn out. I am exhausted myself. She rubs my back with the little energy she has left and I reciprocate. A few minutes later she looks at me and says, "I never do this and it's the first time I have done anything like this and I don't want you to think it's something I usually do." I nod. Not that I care either way.

Her phone is vibrating. It is a friend of hers, asking where she is.

"No, I haven't left. I'm still in the club. I'll come find you," she shouts and hangs up.

"A friend of mine — I better join her."

She embraces me again, adding, "… in a little while."

It is about time we leave the bathroom stall. For a girl who claims to never do anything like this she is surprisingly hard-boiled. (According to girls, no girl ever has a one-night stand or blows some random dude in the club or cheats on her boyfriend.) She coolly walks out of this bathroom stall in the men's room and then proceeds to fix her hair and makeup in front of the mirror, while I wash her dried menstrual blood off my hands. It does not bother her at all that guys are walking in and out. We leave the men's room.

I thought this interaction was over now but then she pulls out her phone again.

"Do you want my number?", she asks.

"Sure."

"You're really fun. Maybe we can hang out again."

We exchange numbers.

"I'm in Berlin for a couple of days. I'm actually checking whether I want to study here."

"Oh! Which universities are you looking at?"

She looks at me. Then, after a pause, she starts laughing.

"You're so funny! No, me and my friends are exploring the city. Universities are all the same anyway."

That is not quite how I see it, but whatever. I smile.

She walks off. I am ready to go home as I am thoroughly exhausted. On the way out, I bump into Orgasms and her friend. I wave goodbye, but she waves me over. She introduces me to her friend, then she gives me a very tight hug. Tonguing her down would have been a bit inappropriate, so we exchange kisses on the cheek.

"Do you have plans for Saturday?", I ask her.

"Nothing in particular yet. Well, you have my number."

I'm off.

❦

I call her on Saturday. She sounds very excited to hear from me but tells me that she cannot talk right now. I take this as a blow-off so I go about my day. About an hour later, however, she is calling me back.

"Listen, Aaron, it was really fun with you."

Uh-oh.

"But I ..., I don't think I can meet you again. I know that if I met up with you, I'd only end up cheating on my boyfriend."

"OK."

"I had such a lot of fun with you, though. No guy has ever made me come like you. I don't think I'll ever forget this."

"Glad you've enjoyed it."

"I did. Good luck and goodbye!"

So that is that. Thank God I did not make her cheat on her boyfriend. I guess for some women it is only cheating if they, while you have your cock in them, say something like, "I'm right now cheating on my boyfriend." Otherwise they are not cheating because they do not have another guy's cock in them *at this very moment*. That's quite a double standard, considering that their boyfriend would get a load of shit if he did as much as glance at another woman. Guys, the takeaway here is that if your girl is having a "girls' night out" or, worse, is on a "fun trip with the ladies," chances are that she cannot wait to gobble down some random dude's cock.

Recruiting a Fuck Buddy

Berlin has a strange party scene. In most Western cities the popular clubs cater to the mainstream: The venues are glitzy, people dress up, and the music consists of the Top 40 played up and down. Alcohol consumption is common, if not rampant. In comparison, in Berlin the most popular places are shady, grimy shit-holes that play techno music. It is the farthest from glitz you can imagine. People do not dress up at all. In fact, plenty dress down. Chicks show up in worn-out second-hand dresses. Guys come in sweatpants. It is ridiculous. People drink alcohol but often only to wash down pills with it. A random sample of one of those clubs would probably reveal that more people are on MDMA or cocaine than buzzed on alcohol.

The trendiest clubs are temporary and are referred to as illegal clubs. It is not illegal to go there. Instead, their owners ignore the laws and operate without either registering their business or without a license to sell alcohol. Some find creative uses of the law, such as a place called Villa, which is housed in a dilapidated old mansion within city boundaries. For all I know, the organizers of that club could be squatters. There, instead of paying a cover charge, you become a temporary member of a non-profit organization for the duration of one night. In Berlin, the city government seems to view laws as a sordid relic of the Nazi era. Otherwise I could not explain all the bullshit I see day in and day out.

That is enough of a prelude.

I have taken it easy for a few days. On Friday I stayed in because I felt too tired. I currently have three fuck buddies and sometimes I just fuck way too much and cannot be bothered to even leave my apartment. Friday was like that. Today is Saturday. I am busy running a few errands and I am drowning in work. I am doing an internship, which I sometimes blow off and think of quitting anyway. Then I do a bit of sport and I have women to fuck. That is my entire week. Going out during the week has been tough. Now that it is Saturday and I have not gone out for about a week, it is high time I get going.

As I am not quite feeling it I text a bunch of my friends for suggestions and ask if they want to tag along. A girl named DRESS, whom you have met before, writes back that she is going to Villa, supposedly the most popular club in town right now. I have only heard of it but never been there. I never felt like going. Quite recently a DJ friend of mine had even put me on the guest list but I got sidetracked and did not show up in the end. Tonight I am going to check out this club.

I show up at around 2 a.m. At the door a bouncer asks me for the password. "The *what*?", I think. I heard some guys in front of me say "thunder heist" or something like that. If I pronounced this like a Londoner the bouncer would not even understand me, so I do my best to ape a strong German accent, butchering the diphthong *th* and pronouncing the vowels in "heist" all wrong. *Ze bounsa* is pleased with my performance and lets me in. I roll my eyes.

Once inside it hardly gets better. As I said before, the club is in a run-down mansion. There are two dance floors, two bars, and two smokers' areas. In order to be more authentic, I suppose, the toilets are kept in a complete mess. Somebody has presumably kicked a urinal off the wall and the pipe has been amateurishly plugged. I check out the bathroom stalls. A few of them cannot be locked. In others the toilet seats are missing. The ones the owners of Villa are surely most proud of have toilets that cannot be flushed. I am pretty grossed out by this place and I regret having become a temporary non-voting member of the non-profit organization — good one! — that runs it.

I walk around some more. The place is slowly filling up. Then I hear someone shout, "Aaron, Aaron! Asshole Aaron!" I look up. It is Dress who is running toward me with her arms stretched out. We have fun catching up. She probes if I have gotten laid recently. I ask her if she has breathed recently. If I tell her any specifics she will only want to hear more. In particular, she is very eager to learn about what other girls do in bed and whether some chick has done something I particularly liked. Well, nobody can say that she does not like to learn anything, unlike her spotty educational record may suggest.[1]

After a while I wish Dress good luck getting picked up. I am on my way again. There are plenty of women in the venue but I do not like the vibe of the place. That

---

[1] In case you are curious what becomes of such women: Dress rode the cock carousel until her early 30s. She was not super hot but certainly good-looking enough to get plenty of male attention. The party ended after getting pregnant by some random dude who quickly disappeared. Yet, she wanted to keep the kid. A few years later another random guy knocked her up. History repeated itself: He left; she kept the kid. In the end she turned into a welfare queen as she was unemployable and missed her chance to marry a good provider when she was young. In other countries or even other parts of Germany she would likely be worse off. However, in Berlin a single mom with two kids makes bank. I looked into the numbers once. It is downright sickening.

is a bit of a shame because as I am walking around I notice about a handful of women who are obviously interested in me, based on their signals: glancing over, rubbing their tits against me as I walk past, or dancing in front of me, shaking their ass invitingly.

There is, of course, no air-conditioning. The air quality is also quite poor. To get some respite I take my T-shirt off but keep on my scarf. I have more body fat than Brad Pitt in Fight Club but also more muscle mass. Chicks dig how I look. In fact, I am used to women coming up to me to touch my arms, pecs or abs, or ask if they can touch me. They also like squeezing my bulging veins. Occasionally I get my crotch grabbed. I would have no problem with that if all women in the world were beautiful. Alas, that is not the case. Anyway, my scarf is annoying me, so I take it off, too. Now I am the only guy who is dancing half-naked in the venue. It takes only a moment for some girl to awkwardly dance in front of me. I pull her in. Moments later she is running her hands down my sweaty pecs and abs. She is licking her lips. Her girlfriends panic as they see this and then the mother hen drags her off.

I shrug and keep dancing. Now I feel two fingers running down my spine. I turn around — it is a dude! He ignores the expression of consternation on my face and leans in to kiss me. I turn my head and put my right arm to fend him off, which he misinterprets as an invitation to suck on my left earlobe. That is enough! I push him away with both hands as I tell him to fuck off. "Sorry. I didn't think you're so uptight," he wails. I clench my fists and assume a fighting stance. Drunk gay men can be a pest. He gets the hint and buggers off.

The music is slowly getting better but this does not last long because some sucky live act comes on, which kills the mood. Now people are just watching the band. As I walk around some more I notice TALLBLONDE in the crowd. She played a very minor role in *Sleazy Stories II*. It seems that she still has the hots for me. She is with some dude and making out with him, but she is also trying to make eye contact with me. I walk over to her, just to see what would happen. She breaks the make out, turns away from her guy and stares at me. As I walk past we just exchange a brief "hi," but she furtively grabs my crotch and tugs it. There might be some other time to pick her up.

The live band has stopped playing; people start dancing again. It is time to enter the fray once more. Some cute girl looks at me and gives me a sexy smile. Then she looks up and down my naked upper body. I walk up to her. As I am about to take her hand I feel a big, strong hand on my neck that is pulling me sideways. I turn around. It is a huge dude.

"Put your clothes on again! The people here don't really like that," he barks.

"It doesn't seem like that at all to me. Besides, do I look like I give a fuck?"

His grip on my neck is getting firmer.

"Listen, jerk-off, I'm not just anybody in this club. I'm a bouncer. If you don't put your clothes back on like right fucking now, it'll be my pleasure to kick you out."

This is a good argument whose validity I acknowledge. I dress myself again. Also, it is around 5 a.m. and I am way too stingy to now pay ten euros or so at some other place. Had it been earlier in the night I might have left the venue as I do not particularly like it here anyway. Yet, I am a sucker for the sunk-cost fallacy.

With my T-shirt back on I am sweating a lot more. Some dude approaches me and asks me something. I do not understand a single word. Then I see a cute girl next to me and ask her how she is doing. The dude backs off. I do not really get anywhere with that chick but at least that was an elegant way to get rid off that guy. Now a girl turns around and blurts out, "I have forgotten my phone number. Can I have yours?"

Let us call her PHONEY. I have a befuddled look on my face as I try to process this interaction. She is really good-looking, but she seems quite awkward. I can tell that she expects an immediate reaction, which she does not get from me. Thus, she looks embarrassed and turns away. How about you give me more than two seconds to come up with a response to your surprise attack, slut? Anyway, that interaction was pretty odd. I take a piss and as I come back some other guy talks to the cutie who had just stumped me. Now I notice that her friends are standing next to me. One of them winks at me.

I say to her, "I get it: You're trying to hook up your friend."

"True. But he actually approached her and unlike you he didn't just walk off."

I sense some passive-aggressiveness. PHONEY had hurriedly turned away because she was unable to deal with a pause. It seems she expected me to respond immediately after she had blurted out her corny pick-up line. Anyway, her friend continues, "It's a shame because we had chosen you for her but you didn't want her."

"She's very attractive, but we didn't have a good vibe. Sorry, can't help it."

She did not like that response and gives me a dirty look. Moments later she is gone.

I lean against the wall, minding my own business. After a few minutes a girl who is giving off a really horny vibe comes up to me.

She says, "What are you doing here?"

I put my hand on her lower back and pull her in as I say, "Nothing much. Just hanging out."

"You so look like some movie star!"

"Let me guess: Adrien Brody?" (I get this a lot.)

"No, not him. It's ...."

I do not understand the name. After asking her to repeat it I still do not, so I just say, "Thank you, that's sweet of you."

In the corner of my eye I notice that PHONEY and her friends are observing me. That guy she was talking to has disappeared already. Her two friends are likewise quite interested in what is going down, but PHONEY shyly averts her gaze after briefly making eye contact with me.

My hand is on that woman's waist. Now I put it on her lower back and push her toward me so that her body is pressing against mine. There is quite some sexual energy unfolding. After some meaningless banter I think that I should better go for the make out, so I slowly lean in. Our lips touch but she stops.

"Do you want to make out that quickly?"

"I wouldn't mind if I was already fucking you."

I look into her eyes with a deadpan expression on my face. She grabs my ass. I grab hers. Our lips are millimeters apart. Yet, I do not give in because I can handle the sexual tension. So can she, incidentally. Now some guy comes over and meekly asks what she is doing. She introduces him to me, then sends him away.

"I'm having an affair with him, but it's nothing serious," I learn.

"I bet he has no idea how to handle a woman like you."

"Um, yes, but it's not just that. He's also so needy and insecure."

"Let's sit down somewhere."

I take her hand and lead her to a sofa. She sits down next to me and snuggles up to me, but I lift her up and put her on my lap. She wraps her arms around me. We talk about random things while caressing each other. In between we make out. Her simp of a lover comes over once again, with a hunched back and his shoulders curled forward. This time he lasts only marginally longer. It seems she has trained him like a dog. Why is he even going out with her if she is free to flirt with other guys? Also, at no point did he challenge me. He succumbed to me right off the bat. I think part of the reason this woman is flirting with me is to test his mettle and he is failing miserably.

This chick is now sharing sex stories. I have a few up my sleeve as well. (If I did not write any of them down, it would be one messy blur but I can recall recent ones quite well.) Her crowning achievement is a threesome with two homosexuals. She is mightily proud of getting two faggots to fuck her. If dykes were hot, the inverse would be a badge of honor for guys as well.[2]

"How about I fuck you in the bathroom?", I suggest.

She grabs my crotch, "It's not that I don't like the idea of you fucking me, but the bathroom stalls in this place are gross."

That is not an option. Neither was going to her place as she lives quite far outside the city center of Berlin. She does not want to come home with me either because "that guy is driving me and I have some things at his place." We exchange contact details and arrange to meet in the coming week. I say goodbye to her with a heavy make out. As I slide one hand into her bra and squeeze her shapely breasts she taps my crotch, trying to identify where my hard cock is. After this keen explorer has discovered its location she grabs and tugs it. As there is the risk that she will make me jizz my pants (no, seriously, I'm pretty turned on), I grab both her wrists, take them with one hand, push them back

---

[2] I am using terms like "faggot" and "dyke" as a sign of respect. In fact, I had a gay flatmate for some time from whom I have learned a lot about this subculture. (I hope you're doing well, P.!) Through him I learned that supposedly derogatory terms are often used as a badge of honor. If he had a few beers too many he would tell you that he is "really proud to be a faggot" and comment on the "great sodomists who built Western culture." Did you know that Leonardo Da Vinci was gay? Neither did I.

over her head and tongue her down while rubbing her crotch with my other hand. She is moaning. Then I get up.

"I'll see you next week," I say.

"Yeah, see you, Casanova! I'm looking forward to it."

My night at Villa was not over at that point. However, I would like to continue with talking about the subsequent encounter with that girl as it does not warrant its own chapter.

❦

We exchanged a couple of text messages and met up on Tuesday at around 8 p.m. I told her to meet me at a station called Bernauer Strasse, which has the double benefit of being close to a park, Mauerpark, and within walking distance to my place. We meet at the station. She greets me by tonguing me down. We are off to a good start. As the weather is not too bad I brought a blanket with me as well as a bottle of red wine. We are off to Mauerpark, holding hands and chatting about random stuff. Then she stops me, grabs my neck, gets on her toes and shoves her tongue in her mouth. We make out.

"I have been fantasizing about meeting you again," she says.

"Happy to hear that," I respond with a smirk and slap her ass.

A few minutes later we are at Mauerpark, close to a hedge. I spread the blanket on the grass and we sit down. I uncork the bottle of wine I brought with me. I normally do not drink so I announce that she has to take care of most of it. She takes the bottle and finishes about a third of it, drinking from the bottle instead of the cheap paper cups I brought. That is a start! I take a sip but from a cup because I am more cultured than this tattooed piece of trash.

She climbs on my lap. Moments later she is kissing me and rubbing my crotch.

"You know, that's not a bad idea," I say to her as I shove my hand into her tight jeans and grab her pussy. Things are getting hot and heavy. To give us some privacy I wrap the blanket around us.

"I know you want to fuck me," she says.

I do not say anything in return. Instead, I unzip her jeans, pull them halfway down her thighs and ram my middle finger up her pussy.

"Ooohh!", she moans.

She grabs my hair and pulls it. I gently choke her. She retaliates by playfully slapping me in the face. I throw her off me and pin her down by pressing her wrists into the grass.

"Fuck me, big boy!", she whispers.

I fish for a condom. I hold it in front of her mouth and she uses her teeth to tear it open. Moments later the condom is on my cock. She is on her back. I tease her by rubbing my cock over her pussy. She is not having any of it, so she grabs it and steers it into her dripping wet hole. Because we are in public I can obviously not cause too much attention, but there are barely any people around anyway. I fuck her slowly, which is not good enough for her.

"Fuck me harder, come on!", she demands.

I pull her hair. Now I sink my teeth into her neck. She moans. Simultaneously, she impatiently pushes her pelvis up rhythmically.

"How about you fuck me properly, little boy?"

I chuckle. How do I get out of that? I take a look around. Because I cannot see any people anywhere I get on my knees, put her ankles on my shoulders, and ram her really hard for a few good thrusts. She moans very loudly, so I have to cover her mouth with my hand.

"Mm–uh, Mm–uh," she utters as she is sucking on my middle, index and little finger. I give her one last hard thrust. Then I pull out and pull the condom off.

"Why do you stop? You weren't done yet."

"Neither were you. We're going to my place now."

Her response to that is a very wide smile, accompanied by a lustful look. We fix our clothes and leave the park.

❦

We are at my place in Prenzlauer Berg. I open the door and shoo her in. My room is the first one to the left in the hallway. From the looks of it, at least one of my flatmates is home too. Well, now is not the time to be considerate of them. I kick off my shoes. She keeps hers on. I open the door to my room, slap and grab her ass, and steer her in. In my room there is a wardrobe to the right, a desk with a chair to the left, and the bed at the end. I do not think we are going to make it into bed.

I close the door behind me. As I turn around she wraps her arms around me and kisses me. We briefly make out, but then I turn her around, bend her over my desk and rub her pussy. I have one hand on her pussy; the other is on her lower back. Where did I put my condoms? Right, there is a box on the nightstand. I step sideways, grab the box, and pull out a condom.

She turns around, unbuckles my belt, unzips my pants and pulls them down.

"I'll help you with that," she says as she reaches into my boxers and pulls my cock out. She's squatting down and takes my cock into her mouth. I'm pleased with her because she is sucking it really well. I grab the back of her head and yank it back and forth. The tip of my cock hits the back of her throat.

I pull her off. With her mouth agape she is taking some deep breaths.

"Time to fuck," I say, as I roll the condom over my cock and grab my shaft. She is getting up.

"Turn around!", I command her.

She smiles and bends forward. I pull her jeans down to her knees and warm her up with two fingers in her pussy, then they have to make way for my hard cock. As I am so horny I just jackhammer her. In terms of height, she is a really good match for my desk. I grab her hair and pull her head back with one hand, with the other I grab her waist and pull her in as I ram my cock into her.

"Aaahhhh! Aaaahhhhh!", she moans loudly and rhythmically.

For added effect she hits my desk with her flat hand intermittently. That probably hurts a little bit. I keep ramming her, but to make it even more fun, I stuff my right middle finger into her asshole. Now I am pounding her pussy slowly.

"Aahh! Aahhh! Aaahh!", she moans.

I pull my middle finger out, put some lube on my right

thumb and stretch out her asshole as I am pounding her. Then I surprise her by putting my cock in her butt.

"Aaaahhhhhhhh!"

She probably saw this coming.

Her asshole is tight, so I end up blowing a load quickly. I pull out and pant heavily. She is panting, too. She turns her head around and looks at me.

"That was great!", she whispers.

"I just wanted to fuck you. I really needed that."

I am still panting.

She turns around, pulls the condom off and throws it into the trash bin.

"You don't mind me cleaning up, do you?", she says.

I nod while I am panting.

She moves on to licking my cock and sucking on it gently. In between, she is making sexy "Mmm!"-sounds. She is doing a really good job.

"Let me return the favor," I say as lift her up and throw her onto my bed. I shove the index and middle finger of my left hand into her mouth. She quickly deepthroats them and moves her tongue over them. I pull my fingers out and put them into her pussy. With my other hand I hold her down while I massage one of her breasts but quickly give her my left thumb to suck on. Meanwhile, I am massaging her G-spot.

"Ooohh, ooooohhh!", she moans.

After not much more than a minute she comes. I drop down next to her. She turns around and snuggles up to me. After she has finished panting she whispers in my ear, "That was really great!"

I doze off. When I open my eyes again, she is dozing as well. It is around midnight. That is just fucking fantastic! She has to go. I gently shake her.

"Huh?", she utters.

"It's really late. I think you should head home."

"How late is it?"

"Past midnight."

"Shit! I'm not going to get home anymore."

I look at her.

"Um," she says, looking at me. Now she is pouting.

"Whatever. I'll make an exception. You can sleep on the couch in the living room."

"What?"

"I'm kidding. You can sleep in my bed, but don't think that you're now my girlfriend."

She nods.

I get up, disappear to the bathroom and ready myself for bed. After I have returned she heads to the bathroom. A few minutes later she is back. She kisses me and then we are making out again. I taste toothpaste.

"Did you bring your toothbrush?", I ask.

"Um, actually, I have my toothbrush in my handbag, but there is a mug with your name in the bathroom so I took yours."

"Okay."

I find that a bit gross and make a mental note to throw out my toothbrush in the morning. Before I can say anything about this to her, her tongue is in my mouth again. I break the make out.

"It's probably too much information and don't let this get to your head. The last chick I fucked — I closed my eyes and imagined that I'm fucking you instead."

"Really?", she squeaks giddily.

"Yup."

"When was that?"

"Saturday."

"What, you met another girl that night — and fucked her?"

"You made me so horny. What was I supposed to do?"

She laughs and adds, "I think you're funny."

"Actually, the guy you saw me with on Saturday ...."

"Uh-uh?"

"I'm no longer seeing him. I didn't want to have sex with him anymore."

I look at her. She looks at me.

We kiss gently, then passionately and deeply. Soon afterward we fall asleep. She is cuddling up to me.

The next morning I am late for work because I just had to bust a nut in her. I do not care for my internship or that industry anymore anyway, so it does not matter. I swagger into the office, not giving a fuck. My colleagues have written me off already, despite me being more productive than half the full-timers in my group. They later told me that I am "not a team player." That's what you get if you do not let your back-stabbing female colleagues take credit for your work.

You may wonder what happened to that chick. That's a simple story: I fucked her on and off for a few months. Eventually she ghosted on me. I assume she simply found another boyfriend. If it is not that then she likely got tired of my supposed commitment phobia.

"But you have to call me the next day!"

That I would eventually fuck the girl the last chapter ended with was of course not clear to me after my interaction with her in the club. Yet, she had managed to make me really horny. I wanted to get laid, if only to get rid of my blue balls. Let's continue from that point onward.

I head back to the dance floor and loosen my shoulders. I slowly get into the beat and start moving my body. A blonde girl with an expensive handbag — I have no idea whether it is an original — looks at me, smiles, and mirrors my movements. I smile back, then I poke her tummy. She laughs and pokes me back. There is quite some zest in this woman! I move closer, grab her waist with both hands, and pull her in. She throws her arms around me and grinds her pussy against my thigh. I think my search is over already. Well, it is quite late, so it is no longer the time to be too picky. She is not super-hot. I would rate her a decent 7 to 8, but closer to a 7. According to my aching balls she will do for tonight.

I go for the kiss. We are making out. Done. After a few seconds she abruptly and awkwardly breaks the make out. It is as if she realized that she has broken one of her rules because first she went in really passionately but then she hastily retracted. She looks at me in a be-fuddled manner. Then she smiles and leans in again. We make out once more. Whatever internal dialogue she may have had seems to have concluded in my favor. She is now getting quite aggressive, grabbing my hair with her petite fingers and pulling it while she is grind-ing her pussy against my leg. I up the ante by grabbing her crotch and rubbing her pussy. She is pretty slen-der, so I am probably hitting her like a truck with my patented grab-and-rub move.

"Mmmhh," she moans.

I take her hand and drag her off the dance floor. We make our way through the crowd. Obviously, I lead her to the bathroom stalls. We are inside the men's re-stroom, in front of the stalls. It is pretty busy in here. I push her against the wall and shove my tongue down her throat. Her physiology is completely changed. It is as if she has been readying herself for penetration. She does not hold back at all. I throw in some crotch rubbing and neck biting before I pull back.

"You're way too aggressive," she says.

"You realize that I just pulled back, don't you?"

"Yeah, but you only do this to tease me," she says, and rubs my crotch, looking for my hard cock. She quickly finds it and tugs it. I grab her hair, yank her head back and bite her neck hard.

"Ouch!", she shrieks.

"Was this too much for you?"

"No."

She sternly looks at me, then she grabs my hair. The other hand is under my T-shirt, scratching my back. At the same time she bites my neck. I grab her head again and pull her off. Then I briefly bite her. My lips brush against her ear. "I'm quite aggressive, but I can also be gentle," I whisper and proceed to softly kiss her neck. She wraps her arms around my neck in response. I would say she is melting.

"You're good at this. You're really good at this," she breathes.

One of the stalls opens. I take her hand and try dragging her in. She resists.

"Come on."

"Nuh-uh!"

She does not like the idea. As we are at an impasse I shove her against the wall and make out with her.

"I'm long past doing such things," she claims.

Whenever I hear something like this from a younger woman, I tend to assume that she has not done anything remotely like having sex in a stall with a complete stranger. With older ones who are nearing 30 it could well be that they want to move on from banging dudes in bathroom stalls and instead pretend to have morals. Anyway, I make out some more with her, with the goal of trying again later. She is not having any of it.

"I like you, but we'd have to go somewhere else," she protests.

"Sure. Where do you live?"

"Not gonna tell you," she says and winks.

I laugh.

"Where do you live?", she wants to know.

"Prenzlauer Berg, around Schönhauser Allee."

"Did you just say Schönhauser Allee?"

"Yup."

"You're kidding me, right?"

"I'm not."

"Come on, you can't seriously live there."

That part of Berlin is seen as pretentious and superficial. In any well-run city it would be the scruffy part of town, but in Berlin any district in which trash does not pile up two feet high on the pavement is considered snobbish. I do not want to discuss this topic rationally with her, so I tongue her down again. I put her hand on my crotch. She rubs it incompetently at first. Then her fingers make their way up to my belt and under my T-shirt. Moments later I feel three fingertips making their way slowly into my pants. I unbuckle my belt to make her job easier. She puts her other hand on mine and says, "We shouldn't go that far."

We are making out again. Meanwhile, she caresses the pubic hair above my cock awkwardly with her fingertips.

"Okay, let's dance some more," she suggests.

We leave the bathroom. I think we should get out of this club. The dance floor is on the way to the exit anyway.

"Wait, where is my friend? She must be here somewhere."

I smirk, "She probably left because she felt that you're in good hands now."

She smiles. Now she is looking around, looking for her friend. She looks a bit lost. Then some dude walks over, apparently an acquaintance. They briefly talk to each other while she keeps holding my hand. He walks off.

"Actually, you were right. She left the place already."

I nod and add, "OK. Let's get out of here."

She looks me deep in the eyes. I do not flinch. After a long five seconds or so she says, "OK."

We get our jackets and head off. As we make our way down from the club to the streets she says two or three times, "But you have to call me the next day!" She wants more than a mere one-night stand. If she is not spectacular in bed her chances are slim. I would not at all be surprised if she is used to getting pumped and dumped. She is exactly the kind of chick you go for if you did not manage to pull any of the really hot ones. That is not to say that she is not attractive. She is just not the kind of girl you want to fuck repeatedly because there are plenty of hotter ones around. Instead, she is the kind of girl to get your rocks off with in a pinch.

"So, where do you live?", I ask her.

"I'm not going to tell you."

"No problem. We're going to my place then."

"No way! I don't want to be seen anywhere around fucking Schönhauser Allee."

This again! I am holding both her hands.

"This is silly. I don't even know your name," she says.

After exchanging our names we make out passionately again.

"My place is kind of a mess, to be honest," I say to her.

She does not say anything for a while, then she excitedly shrieks, "Cab, cab!"

A cab stops.

"Is this our cab?", she asks.

"Sure is."

Because of her hesitating, another couple reaches the cab before us. The next cab is coming up, though.

"Let's go to your place," I say.

She does not say anything.

"I'll call you, don't worry," I add.

She looks at me, smiles, and says, "Really?"

We hop into the cab, which takes us to her place. The ride takes a few short minutes. We could have easily walked there. Man, if I were looking for a girlfriend, someone so indecisive and thriftless would not make the cut. The driver stops. She does not flinch at all, seemingly expecting me to pay for it. I pull out a two-euro coin. She is chipping in four euros. I almost feel dirty paying for it. There is hope she is worth two euros.

She is living alone. Her flat is quite small but tidy. I would say it is almost obsessively tidy. I ask her for some water. She comes back from her kitchenette with a glass of water.

"You know, I never ever do anything like this."

"I know."

I used to occasionally say, "Yeah, neither do I," but the last time this made some chick crack up. I do not mind making girls laugh, but right now I want to get my dick wet ASAP instead of having to work around obstacles of my own creation, like wittingly claiming that I am kind of a virgin or some bullshit like that.

She disappears into the bathroom. I sit down on her bed. There is not much else to sit down on as the chair by her desk does not look comfortable and there is no sofa or armchair. It is a pretty spartan place, all things considered. She is coming back from the bathroom and sits down on my lap, straddling me. Now she is gently kissing me, covering my face with sweet little pecks of her lips. Then she stops.

"Why you?", she rhetorically asks.

"Yeah, why always me?", I think. I do not say a word, though.

"I mean, I've spoken with so many guys in the club, but why was it you in the end?"

"Your other suitors were probably all incompetent and didn't know how to get a girl."

"Yeah, probably."

She leans in. We kiss again.

Well, that's all there really was to it. Now some of you may think that it's amazing that I can go out and consistently pull chicks. But quite often it's only great in theory. Sure, some girls are amazing in the sack. It is quite rare to find those. The girl I was with that night, though, does not belong to that category.

What, you want me to tell you about a shitty lay? Alright, if you insist — but do not bitch about it afterward!

Back to the story:

"Can you undress?", she asks.

"Are we in a particular hurry?"

"No, but I want to turn the lights off."

"You want to turn the lights off?"

"I don't like doing it with the lights on."

I do not often encounter this anymore. I guess I bump into too many hard-boiled sluts. Anyway, I get out of my clothes. Meanwhile, she opens the drawer of her nightstand and produces a tea light. She also pulls out a pyramid made of stained glass into which she slides the tea light after lighting it. After turning off the lights of her room, the red-and-purple-colored glass pyramid sets the mood. I am hoping that this is going to get quite kinky. The atmosphere is how I imagine some cheap Eastern European whore doing business at home in her bedroom would set it.

She leans forward to kiss me. I tackle her playfully. She is on her back. I mount her.

"You're really wild. I like it."

"How about you start with sucking my dick?", I suggest as I'm moving, on my knees, closer to her face.

"I don't really do this," she claims.

I reach behind and put my middle finger in her pussy. She gets a nice massage. Now she is looking at me, her eyes burning with lust. She opens her mouth but does not moan. She is just breathing more heavily.

"Let's try that again," I say as I put my fully erect dick in her mouth.

She is working on it but she totally sucks at it, pun intended. My dick is getting softer, not harder. We are not off to a good start here. Her tits look pretty great, though. They are small and firm and nicely shaped. I spit into my hand, rub the spit over her tits, put my cock in between them and titty-fuck her. Judging from the look on her face, she is not getting turned on by this at all.

"Eww, I don't like that! Please do something else," I hear her say.

This is not a lot of fun for me. You really do not want to get that kind of discouraging feedback while you are getting down to it. Her pussy is still pretty wet, so I do not see a fundamental problem with her being a bit uptight. I stroke my dick with the intention of getting harder so that I finally get to fuck her. Because she does not like being relegated to a passive role, she sits up, grabs my dick and whacks it. Being neither able to hold a steady rhythm nor grip it well, this is likewise pathetic. My boner is gone. I am getting a bit pissed off here.

I push her down on the bed again and finger her. She does not moan and does not say anything either. Yet, she is getting pretty into it. The look in her eyes and her half-open mouth tell me that she likes what I am doing. With my other hand I am whacking myself to get hard. This does not take long because her great body looks even hotter when she is squirming. If her face wasn't that plain she would be a serious contender in the sexual arena. Her pussy feels tight. Now it is time to stretch her out a bit with my big cock. I am reaching over to the chair by the table near her bed and pull a condom as well as a bottle of lube out of the inner pocket of my fancy sports coat.

The condom is on my cock.

"What are you doing?", she inquires.

"Nothing," I say as I lube my cock.

"Are you kidding me? You're going out with a bottle of lube in your jacket? What kind of guy are you?", she asks and giggles.

"You'll see."

I am on top, whacking myself with one hand. With the other I support myself as I lower myself on her and kiss her. We kiss passionately. She grabs my balls and tugs them. Now I am getting really impatient. I enter her with one hard thrust. She opens her mouth, closes her eyes, and yanks her head back. I am pounding her. Her mouth is open but there are no sounds coming out of it. Whatever. I just keep pounding her, slowly and steadily. She does not show much of a reaction. After a few minutes of this I am getting tired of it and pull out. I grab her waist and want to pull her over. Immediately, her hands are on my wrists.

"What are you doing?", she wants to know.

"Oh, you'll see."

"No, seriously, I only like it when I'm on my back."

Is she joking? I want to grab her again to turn her over, but she is tensing up.

"No, I really don't feel comfortable doing it any other way."

Because I am not really in the mood anymore, I consider dressing myself and heading home.

"Please, can't you just continue with what you've done before? It was really nice."

She does have a damn fine body, though. I am not going to argue with that. She is playfully caressing her breasts, which gets me horny again. I swap condoms and continue where I had left off. She closes her eyes and gasps for air. I find my rhythm, keep pounding her nice and steady, and think I am going to blow a load in her. As I am not close yet I keep pounding her, but more vigorously. I'm pounding her faster. I'm going to get there! Then she panics, gets up, and stops me when I am at the apex of the thrusting motion. I was preparing myself for the grand finale, yet she holds me back.

"No, don't! Don't come inside of me," she pleads.

It is probably not a good idea arguing about that. I pull out. She quickly pulls the condom off and jerks me. From the look on her face she is really horny. I wanted to finish with a BJ, but instead she jerks me off, pointing my dick to her belly button. Given her tight tummy this is a really sexy sight. She is not doing too badly.

"Mmmm!", I say as I erupt.

She presses my dick into her belly button. Afterward she spreads the cum around with the tip of my cock.

I know it sounds odd but it felt really good. If you are not with a young girl who is in shape and has great firm skin it probably does not feel nearly as good. With a woman past 25 or so it is surely a much different experience.

As I now want to give her an orgasm I start working on her, focusing on her clit and G-spot. Her sexy body squirms as my hands work their magic. She is building up quite an orgasm it seems. Her mouth is open but no moans come out.

"Yeah, oh yeah!", I hear.

I am a bit thrown off by this. Instead of moaning she makes the kind of sounds a guy makes when fucking, based on the knowledge I have from me banging chicks and my study of porn.

"Yeah! Yeah, baby!"

This is really creeping me out as I am getting a male porn voice track spoken by a woman.

"Oh yeeeaaaahhh!"

I shudder.

I keep hitting her G-spot. She is sending shivers down my spine as I hear, "Oh yeah, oh yeah! ... Do you like it, baby? ... How's that?"

I'm ravaging her G-spot with my middle and index finger. She is arching her back. She is coming.

"I'm coming! I'm coming!"

Women normally do not say that either.

As a guy you blow your load and that's it, but a chick has this phase where the orgasm dissipates. Again, she does not utter the usual uh's and ah's which are so typical, but a number of yeah's, which eventually taper off. This all feels odd beyond belief. It is freaking me out. My bet is that she just copied the sounds she heard dudes making when they plowed her.

Her performance has been bizarre, but her squirming body with my dried cum on it looks really hot. I decide to give her another orgasm.

"What are you doing? I just came."

"Let me handle this."

"No, seriously, I don't think I can come again so soon."

I start anyway. It takes me a few minutes, but time is passing quickly as I am marveling at her body. My hands are on autopilot. She is coming again and I get the same painful verbal treatment as before. It is just as bad. After a while she is fully relaxed again.

"That was mind-blowing. I had no idea I could come twice in a row."

I nod.

I feel pretty tired, so I want to nap instead of heading home.

"Is it okay if I crash here?", I ask her.

"It's totally cool."

We head to the bathroom together. I hope my dentist will not get too upset about me awkwardly brushing my teeth by putting some toothpaste on my index finger and using it as a brush. She is brushing properly.

Back in bed she is like a kitten, purring and cuddling up to me. There is still my dried cum on her body.

"Don't you want to remove that?"

"No. I like having it there."

We fall asleep.

After a few hours I wake up, with a nice morning boner to boot. She is half asleep, so I kiss her on her lips.

"Are you awake?", I ask.

"Yeah."

I almost chuckle.

"Good," I say and put her hand on my cock.

"Wow, you're so eager!"

I do her again missionary style, but this time I pull out well before I am close to coming. I hop forward and land with my dick in her face. She is taking it into her mouth. She really is not good at sucking dick, so I jerk myself while she does God-knows-what with her mouth and tongue. I'm not feeling much.

"Stick your tongue out," I command her.

She obliges.

I press the tip of my cock against her tongue while I am whacking myself. The extra stimulation is pretty nice and that is not something she can easily fuck up either. Moments later I am about to blow my load. She notices the pre-cum coming out, so she quickly cocks her head up and takes my dick in, wrapping her lips around the tip. I think she is afraid I would give her a nasty facial or jizz straight into her hair.

Afterward I collapse next to her. She is cuddling up to me. I fall asleep again. An hour or two later I wake up again. She is wrapped around me and now she opens her eyes. I give her two more orgasms with my fingers for old time's sake, but eventually it is time for me to leave. Of course, she insists on me taking her number. I have not the slightest doubt that I could see her again and convert her into a fuck buddy or even a girlfriend (yeah, right). But, alas, I would rather not. The first thing I do after leaving her place is delete her phone number. Was she worth two euros? Probably not. She should have paid me.

The Rules Girl

Monday, 1 June, is a public holiday in Germany. To-day is Sunday, 31 May. I have nothing better to do, as usual, so I head out. As I am in the mood for something new or at least for a club I do not normally go to I pick Weekend at Alexanderplatz. This is one of the more mainstream techno clubs in Berlin. It is a pretty nice place, located in a high-rise building. If Berlin were not such an ugly city you would have an impressive view from there as well.

Upon arrival I am greeted by a queue that is easily 100 people deep. Thankfully it is moving quickly. I get a bit annoyed when they charge me 12 euros instead of their usual 8 euros, which is also what they had advertised in their email newsletter. The ditz at the entrance summarizes the situation as follows when I question her: "It's a public holiday and we've got this great DJ." That surely justifies fraudulent advertising and ramping up cover charge by 50 %. I do not like scammers, so I pay but will not go to Weekend much in the future. That is despite the pretty great story that is about to unfold.

I walk in and wonder where the hell I am. I did not get the impression that today's event was marketed as a gay night and the queue outside was also quite mixed. Yet, for some reason the place is swarming with faggots. For those not familiar with this scene I better point out that there is an enormous difference between a club with a large surplus of straight men, which is commonly referred to as a cock farm or sausage fest, and a party with a surplus of gay men. Women do not feel comfortable in the former crowd but in the latter they get pretty horny because on a trendy club night that caters to a gay clientele you will see a lot of objectively very good-looking men. (I have no idea what parties with unattractive gay men are like. They probably party with butch lesbians and feminists.)

It is really crowded in here. It is not an exaggeration to say that this place is packed to the brim. I find it difficult to move through the crowd and have to gently push people to get out of my way. People? Of course I am talking about men because there are not so many women around. The first dance floor is packed and everybody is sweating. I notice a supremely hot girl twisting her body to the music but she is completely zoned out. She ended up dancing in the same spot for hours next to the DJ and a dense crowd of bulky gay men. As she seems more interested in getting attention than hooking up, my dislike of the idea of having to make my way through a sweaty mass of flesh serves as a welcome justification for not bothering to approach her.

As I do not want gay men to press their naked upper body against me, accidentally or otherwise, I quickly seek refuge on the second floor. Yes, you take an elevator to a higher floor! There I find a much more mixed crowd. It is also really packed. I bet they yanked cover charge up once they realized that they are drawing a big crowd tonight. Some of my favorite watering holes are closed tonight, which probably explains why Weekend is the busiest I have ever seen it.

I look around and my eyes are quickly drawn to a really cute girl dancing in the periphery of the dance floor. I shall call her RULES. She is short, petite, has nice big eyes and really great tits. I bet they are fake. (Let me solve the mystery right away: Her tits turned out to be fake.) There is a guy next to her. It is not obvious to me if he is her friend, boyfriend, or just some random loser. Based on her body language and the fact that she made eye contact with me, which she has been holding, he is a non-issue.

I walk up to her. She is flailing her arms around, supposedly to the beat of the music. When I stop in front of her, her arms are in the air. I grab both her wrists with one hand, the other hand I put on her lower back. Holding her like that I pull her in, pressing her body against mine. We are still making piercing eye contact. I lower her body by moving her arms backward, not unlike a lever. At the same time she is grinding her pussy against one of my legs. I keep her bent backward like this and when I release my grip on her wrists she immediately starts exploring my upper body with her little hands, on and in my shirt. Moments later we are making out.

In order to not give her too much of a release for her pent-up sexual energy I break the make out. We dance some more. She keeps pressing her body against mine and grinding her pussy against my leg. In between we make out some more. I am restraining myself. In a shadier club I would now finger her, but Weekend is not as dark as other clubs and it is also a somewhat classier venue. That does not mean that I do not want to push this interaction further. Quite the opposite is true. To get her in the mood I pull her ass cheeks apart to the beat of the music. We make out again.

Now she is looking over to the guy she had been dancing next to earlier. He seems pretty disinterested and is probably gay anyway. Oh, and now another dude joins him and rubs his abs. I do not think I need to describe those two young men fondling each other. RULES is getting quite turned on by the double-whammy of the interaction with me and seeing her gay friends working hard at arousing each other. My boner is only due to her, though.

This being a somewhat classy club, I do not want to pull my dick out on the dance floor or play with her pussy out in the open, so I take her hand in order to drag her off. She holds her ground.

"No, wait!", she says.

She walks to her friends and I tag along. It seems she wants to make use of their counsel. Particularly among younger women it is quite common that her friends have to confirm that the guy she is hooking up with is indeed hot. Her friends smile at me. One of them high-fives me. The other puts on a big grin. He winks at me, then he says to her, "I know what you want to know, but you started this so now you better follow through with it." He laughs and sends her off by flapping his hand. Gays and their limp wrist!

RULES seems pleased. Our planned destination is of course one of the bathroom stalls. They have unisex toilets in this place. On my way to the nearest one I surprise her by lifting her up, pushing her into the wall and tonguing her down mid-air. She moans, puts her hands under my shirt and scratches my back.

Now we are inside the biggest bathroom at Weekend. It is busy. The queue is long. I am not sure whether

I can keep her horny until it is our turn to enter one of the stalls. There are plenty of not overly attractive regular people around, male and female alike. I realize that I have not said a single word to her yet. Let us see for how long I can keep this up.

As there is not much progress I take her to another bathroom, but this one is full of women, which baffles me at first. Then I realize that the other bathroom is not unisex but for men. Women just shamelessly walk in when they feel like it, while almost no guy dares to enter the female bathroom. This is gender equality in action. There is not much progress either. What is worse, the women in here are showing their dislike for RULES. She is good-looking and has a top-shelf man with her. Most of the women in here surely strike out on both counts and are green with envy.

I do not think I am doing myself any favors by stalling, so I decide to look for the most isolated spot inside the venue, keep her horny, and try again for the restrooms once people start to leave. It is around 2:30 a.m. and this club already closes at 5:00 a.m. In about an hour things should be a lot better.

We make our way back to the crowded dance floor. I look around and indeed I spot some unoccupied seats in some corner. I sit down and pull her down on my lap. She wraps her arms around me and tongues me down right away. It is time to up the ante, so I put one hand under her skirt and rub her crotch. As her full breasts have been beckoning me, I pull one out of her top — she is not wearing a bra — and suck on the nipple. She is moaning, moves her hands through my hair and pulls it. She loves what I am doing.

As we have been making such good progress getting to know each other, I unbuckle my belt, unzip my pants and pull my cock out of my boxers. We make out heavily. I want to put one of her hands on my cock. Yet, she is so alert that she grabs my cock and whacks it the moment I have freed it from its prison. Her other hand is still busy with my hair. If I do not stop her, she will surely make me blow a load. As I do not want to settle for a handjob I may as well see if she will blow me right here. I nibble on her earlobe, then lick her ear. I follow this up by whispering into it, "Come on, suck my dick!" It is too loud in here, so I have to repeat it. Now she understands me. She opens her mouth. However, instead of taking my dick like a good girl she has the audacity to speak. She says, "Actually, I am quite the prude. I can't do that."

Given the circumstances, her choice of words does not make a lot of sense. After all, a prude girl probably wants to spend more than half an hour getting to know a guy before playing with his dick. Judging from her behavior I do not at all believe that she is a prude, at least according to my interpretation of that word.

My immediate goal is to break down her resistance, so the obvious next step is going for her pussy. One of my hands climbs up her firm thigh. I even get two fingers into her panties. Yet, I am apparently too close to her labia. She is freaking out a bit and pulls my hand off with both hands. It later turned out that this did not quite mean what I thought it meant. I will keep you in suspense for now, but let me just say that you do not meet many girls with her kind of beliefs. A further hint is that she has no problem with me stimulating her clitoris through the garment of her skirt and, later, her panties. But back to the action!

I reposition her so that she sits next to me. I put an arm around her and exert pressure on her back, indicating that she should put her head in my lap. My cock is still out, by the way. She rests her head in my lap and looks at my erect penis. I take it with one hand and grab the back of her head with the other, intending to put one and one together. She resists. I am walking a thin line here, so I better not push her too much. She sits up again.

"I liked looking at your cock from that angle," she says.

"I would have liked putting my cock into your mouth," I smoothly respond.

She laughs and says, "Don't be ridiculous. We're in the middle of a club."

"We're in a secluded corner. Nobody would notice it

anyway and if they did they wouldn't care. I think it's totally fine if you sucked me off."

Admittedly, that is a rather bold conjecture on my part, but what else am I supposed to do? I try again to make her suck me right here, and again. Both attempts fail. She is getting a bit annoyed by it. "I think I should get back to my friends," she says.

Judging from how she is looking at me and by the fact that one of her hands is under my shirt, clutching my cock, I do not think I have messed up this interaction.

"Let's go somewhere else instead," I suggest.

I get up, put my dick away, and tongue her down. I want to leave the club with her. I take her hand and walk downstairs to the first floor of the club. The closer we get to the exit, the more she resists. Finally, she stops me.

"I know what you're doing. But I don't even know the city. I don't know anybody here and don't know my way around either. We flew into Berlin just two days ago."

"What are you in Berlin for anyway?"

"Oh, my friends and I studied abroad in Europe, but now we're just traveling around before we head back to the States."

"Nice. Where do you study at?"

"Ohio State."

"How is it there?"

"Super fun!"

I need to chuckle but I quickly rub the side of my nose with my opposite thumb, not because my skin is itching but because I do not want her to see my reaction and this looks more natural than covering my mouth with my hand. Ohio State University is a party school. That I am not dealing with a Rhodes Scholar does not surprise me, but she is a cliche.

Her talking about her party school makes her giddy, it seems. She is dancing in front of me. I pick her up and hold her in the air with just one arm. She clutches my cheeks and slowly moves her head toward me with puckered lips. We make out. In between she utters "Mmm!" a few times.

We are at the lower dance floor. By now Weekend has gotten a lot less crowded. What better way to exploit this than by dragging her into a bathroom stall? I first check out the male one, which is still packed. I guess that the faggots are now all fucking each other. The female one on the other hand is not busy at all. There are just two girls in front of us who are waiting for their turn.

RULES protests, "I'm not sure I want to do this."

Instead of saying anything in response I squeeze her ass and tongue her down.

The discrepancy between her words and actions has gotten quite stark. As she tells me, "I'm not going to go in there with you," she is pressing her body against mine, followed by her initiating a make out. I am used to girls telling me that they are "not like other girls", "not one of *that* kind of girls" or that they "never do anything like this," even when they are exactly like all the other girls and thus like *that kind of girls* who eagerly engages in promiscuity. Those women first put up a front and then they passionately make out with you or squat down and readily take your dick. Similarly, RULES tells me that she is not that kind of girl while behaving exactly like that kind of girl. Saying that her words lack persuasive power would be an understatement.

After what feels like ten minutes it is finally our turn. As I open the door of the bathroom stall some gay-looking dude tries jumping the queue and sneak in. I put up an arm to hold him back.

"Sorry, I really have to pee. Can I get in first?", he asks.

I do not answer and instead usher RULES into the bathroom stall.

The gay dude shouts, "Make it quick, please! I gotta pee!"

I lock the door. The moment I turn around she jumps up, wraps her legs around me and shoves her tongue into my mouth. I reach around and rub her crotch. This goes on for just a few moments, but now some asshole starts banging on the door. I do not like external pressure and neither does she. She looks quite uncomfortable indeed. I nonetheless push on.

I pull my cock out and whack myself in front of her. She quickly takes over, puts the other hand on my neck and pulls me toward her. We are making out again. The banging on the door gets louder.

"Hurry up, guys!", someone is yelling.

No, none of this is helping me.

I sit RULES down on the toilet. This one thankfully does not only have a seat attached to it but also a toilet seat cover. I think I mentioned that Weekend is one of the classier clubs in Berlin. I stand in front of her. She still has my cock in her hands. She looks at me, then at my cock, then at me again. It seems I am getting close to some hopefully decent cock-to-mouth action. Those assholes outside are now banging on the door rhythmically. I can make out multiple hands. Is this some kind of riot or what?

She is looking at my dick again.

I hear a crack and now the lock of the door of the bathroom stall gives in. Those motherfuckers really managed to break open the door! The door flings open. RULES panics, gets up, and rushes outside. Thanks, you motherfucking assholes!

Some dude squeezes himself into the bathroom stall. I want to shout at him but I have to hurry after RULES, putting my cock into my boxers, zipping my pants, and fixing my belt on the way. I barely pay any attention to the bystanders. Nonetheless I register that there is once again a queue. I feel like socking one of those assholes, but I have no time for that. I have to take care of that chick.

I have almost caught up to her. She is walking a lot slower already. I grab her wrist; she turns around. I pull her in. We make out. She is panting, but after a while she is calm again. At first she resists my tongue entering her mouth and is a bit tense as well. Yet, she quickly warms to me again. I can tell that she is feeling uncomfortable. Now she opens her mouth.

"That was a bit much. I think I should go back to my friends."

That is not good. That is not good at all. Or is it? She put both hands on my shoulders, stands on her toes, and pulls herself up. We are making out again. "I'm fine now," she says and takes my hand. We walk around the club but have little luck finding her friends. RULES is looking around. Given how short she is this is not a winning strategy.

A tall woman appears to my left, wearing a pretty classy dress that exposes her back. She stares into my eyes. I quickly glance down to the floor. Of course, she is wearing heels. She smiles at me, then she puts her long-drink glass against my lips. Meanwhile, RULES's back is turned against me. She is still looking around. She is also squeezing my hand. I am baffled by how sexually aggressive that other woman is, though. As I feel like experimenting I go for a make out. She gives me a big smile but turns her head away, letting me kiss her cheek and the corner of her lips instead. Then she sucks on my neck. She is clearly into me but I do not think it is wise to jump ship, seeing how far I have progressed with RULES already. I walk away with RULES in tow.

Letting RULES get back to her friends is a bad idea. Instead, I usher her to the nearest sofa. I can tell that she is still really horny. I sit down. She immediately sits down on my lap. It seems she has completely forgotten about her friends. We make out and feel each other up. We are also upping the ante. Within a few minutes, we are biting each other's neck. She is pulling my hair as vigorously as I pull hers. It is clear that I have to take this interaction somewhere else. You really do not want to be the guy she knows basically nothing about when the lights in the club go on, so I ask her a few random questions.

"I have to ask you something," she says after a while.

"Just ask."

"Um, are all German men like you?"

"How am I?", I say with a smirk.

"You know, you're like a real man. You just take whatever you want."

"Yup, I do. No, most German men are absolutely not like me. Just look around! Plenty of guys in here are too busy fucking each other to look for a girl."

She bursts out laughing.

"Guys in the US are pretty shitty with women," she says.

"I can imagine."

"Once I was fooling around with this one guy in bed, and he bumped my head into the wall. It wasn't a big deal but then he apologized over and over and over. You can't imagine what a turn-off this was."

"Sounds horrible."

"Yeah. Our men are basically all wussies."

I do not want to talk too much, so I grab her by her hair at the back of her head and yank it. She lets out a lustful moan. She puts both of her little hands on my chest and says, "You know what, you really are a mysterious, tall, dark-haired stranger."

By now she seems really horny, judging by how she is squirming in my lap. The DJ puts on a track with heavy bass. RULES comments that she really likes that track. I take this as an invitation to grab her head and yank it back and forth to the beat. She smiles at me, winks, and then opens her mouth wide. Now she is vigorously deep-throating an imaginary penis. She totally loves it. Not everyone in the venue does, though. Some random guy shows up next to me, taps me on the shoulder and shouts, "This is not a sex club."

I raise my hand and gesture him to bugger off.

"Show some restraint or leave. You two are making people uncomfortable."

"Help me out here: Who the fuck are you again?"

He does not say anything in response and walks off. This guy does not seem like he is staff or security. He is probably just a frustrated faggot who did not manage to find someone to fuck him in the ass tonight. RULES does not take it quite so well. She is sliding off my lap and cuddles up to me. After a while I pull her into my lap again.

"But weren't we just told not to do this?", she asks.

I do not think it is a good idea to discuss that situation in detail with her, so I tell her, "We can make out. A few couples in here do. I think the problem is that I am not supposed to ram a huge imaginary cock down

88

your throat." She giggles. Then she shoves her tongue into my mouth again.

A little later her friends drop by to check up on her, asking whether everything is alright. I have been treating her well and she is visibly enjoying my company. Thus, her friends have no rational reason to interfere. Because they are gay and male they also do not have any reason to be particularly jealous, which can be an issue with female friends of a girl you want to pull.

It is quite late. In fact, it is getting close to 5 a.m. I have more or less given up on the thought of getting my rocks off inside the club. That does not mean that I will not try to get laid the old-fashioned way. She tells me that she is staying with the friends I had just met and that tomorrow they will move to a different apartment, which they have rented together. I do not see how this would prevent her from coming back to my place. I take her hand and lead her off.

"Where are you taking me?", she asks.

I do not answer.

We are now on the ground floor in the building, where the coat check of Weekend is located. The queue there is enormously long, which is not surprising since it is close to closing time and people who go out a lot are familiar with the problem of wanting to leave when everyone else does, too, so they rather not wait until the lights go on before heading off. Of course, this hardly solves their problem. They just end up waiting a little bit less. Instead, they should have left an hour ago already.

"Get your stuff," I tell her.

"I don't want to leave my friends behind."

I try again, but she does not budge. Not even after pushing her into the wall and tonguing her down is she verbally agreeing to leave with me. Well, the verbal agreement is optional. She is walking back to the elevator, which leads to the dance floors. I am not ready to give up yet. Walking off right now would be stupid. I know that she wants my dick. Seeing how many people are now waiting to collect their coat I conclude that we should have much less of a problem finding an unoccupied bathroom stall.

First we sit down some more, cuddle, and make out. I pull out my phone to get her contact details, just in case. Meanwhile, she drops that she does not want to have a one-night stand.

"I can't go home with you. It's not just that I don't really know my way around Berlin, it's also against the rules."

"What rules are you talking about?"

"Well, my rules, you know?"

I nod.

"Also, I don't really know you," she adds.

"What are you talking about? We've spent hours together."

She giggles.

"Actually, that kind of makes sense. I can't say that I don't know you."

"See."

"But ...."

"Well, we don't even really know ourselves, so I don't think that's a good standard," I say and inwardly cringe.

"That's kind of deep."

(It is not. It is akin to the vapid bullshit you hear from students in the humanities.")

I lean in to kiss her. We are making out again.

"You do like cock, don't you?", I ask her with a smirk.

"Don't be silly!", she says and laughs.

Her mouth is quite small but she has full luscious lips, so I drop, "Your mouth is probably too small for my cock anyway," with a deadpan expression on my face.

She giggles.

"I don't know about that, but I like giving head. But I don't always like it. I have to kind of be in a generous mood."

I laugh.

"You know, in my experience girls like giving head as much as guys like getting it," I say.

This is bullshit. Some girls do but certainly not all. I just wanted to see how she reacts to it. Also, it is good to set an ideal for her to strive toward. There is another aspect: I am sure some girls like giving head, but not all of them are that good at it, which causes the guys on the receiving end to not enjoy it much. At the extreme, I would say that every girl who gives shitty head because she is using teeth likes that more than the guy who is getting his cock teethed. The latter most certainly no guy likes. But let us get back to the conversation.

"For me, it all depends on how much I like the guy. But I also have to really know someone."

By now I suspect that she is just cock-teasing me. I pull her in, make out with her, and look her straight in the eyes. I say, "The least you could do is whack me off."

She does not flinch at all.

I take her hand and lead her to the toilets again. I recall that Weekend has three toilet areas. So far I have just checked out two together with her. However, there is a third one, which consists of just two stalls. It is upstairs in the smokers' lounge. This probably would have been the best choice all along.

There is only one stall for each sex and there are hardly any people around anymore anyway. The stall in the men's restroom is occupied, but there is nobody else in there. In the women's restroom, the stall is also occupied and four or five women are gathering around the mirror, brushing up their makeup. I take her back to the men's bathroom.

"I won't do anything with you," she says.

That is of course nonsense.

A dude exits the stall. I usher RULES in. The dark blue light in this stall is pretty cool and almost seductive. I put her through the program: making out, crotch rubbing, putting my cock in her hand. She eagerly whacks it. Then I put her other hand on it as well. Because her hands are so small, this is a really cool moment. She is staring at me with her big eyes while whacking me, which looks as if she is entranced by touching my hard cock. I sit her down on the toilet. Oh, this one also has a toilet seat and toilet seat cover. It is pretty clean. Man, this one almost meets the standard of a cheap hotel!

Someone is knocking on the door. This is really not my day.

"Is somebody in here? We are closing this area shortly. It's almost 5 a.m."

I shout back, "Just give me a few minutes! I am almost

done here."

If he only knew what I am referring to.

RULES is busy whacking my cock. I put one hand on the back of her head and gently push it forward.

"Now suck it!"

She looks up to me but does not respond. Instead, she keeps whacking it. I am getting really hard. There is no reason to wait anymore.

"Come on, suck it!"

She starts by licking the glans and tickling the frenulum with her tongue. This goes on for a while. Eventually she moves on to licking all over the tip of my cock, putting her lips on it and sucking it. I gently take one of her hands off my cock and say, "Take it in deeper!"

She looks at me. Then she takes her other hand off my cock — and slowly puts it in all the way. Due to how small her head is my cock looks enormous in comparison, which I find strangely arousing. She is deepthroating me like a pro. I am really blown away by how good she is. Much sooner than I would have liked my cock starts throbbing. I do not want to restrain myself.

"I'll come in your mouth," I say.

That was a mistake. She quickly takes my cock out of her mouth, yanks it sideways, and looks the other way. She literally lets me stand there with my erect cock.

Well, I am really close to coming, so I stroke myself for a few seconds and tell her to watch me come. She shyly glances at my cock. I am shooting a wad. I have some cum on my index finger, so I put it close to her mouth. She immediately sucks on my finger. Then she realizes that she has just tasted my cum. This makes her flinch, but she still swallows it. She smiles at me. I smile back at her.

We leave the bathroom stall. Afterward, we sit down on the first sofa we come across. More and more people are leaving the club. We just sit there, caressing each other. She is cuddling up to me like there is no tomorrow. Getting me off seems to have been quite the bonding experience for her.

I get the idea of fingering her for a bit, which she does not like at all. This time she lets me touch her labia, but as soon as I want to enter, she panics and pulls my hand out of her pants again.

"What are you doing? I have morals, don't you have morals, too?", she says.

I look at her with a blank expression on my face.

"You know, there are rules which you have to follow," she adds.

"Rules are arbitrary. I prefer making my own."

I pull her in and made out with her again.

At around 5:15 a.m., well after closing time, a security guy walks up to us and tells us to leave. On the way out, we bump into her two gay friends again. They want to head to another club. She is up for it.

"Do you want to come along?", she asks.

"I rather just go home and rest. I'm really tired."

"Sure," she says, giving me a wide, sexy smile. Then she winks.

❦

You may wonder what her rules were. There were just a few. She was in Berlin for about two more weeks and she visited me a few times. She was happy to blow me and from the second blowjob onward she also eagerly swallowed. I was allowed to touch her clitoris and get her off this way. She wanted me to lick her clit but that struck me as a risky proposition. Her pussy was off-limits, though. It was off-limits for every part of my body: tongue, fingers, penis. To make up for that, she was happy to tell me that I can fuck her in the ass all I want. She theorized that she is able to retain her virginity this way.

I asked her how she came up with her rules. It was simply what she thought a "good, religious girl" could do. In fact, she insisted that her approach was "the best of both worlds," because it allowed her to keep her virginity while she still got to experience premarital sex. She was aware that some men value a low partner count or even virginity very highly and it was her goal to find a husband who would provide very well for her. Consequently, she saw her "virginity" as a golden ticket to a life as a pampered housewife.

I did not dare to point out to her that men who want a virginal wife want someone who has not been intimate with anyone before in any imaginable way and not some garden-variety slut who thinks that letting guys fuck them in the ass means that they have found a smart workaround that lets them have their cake and eat it, too. Anybody who puts it in her mouth or her butt may not count for her, but I do not think this is how guys would see it. I have no reason to complain because her other two holes served me very well. Yet, I wonder what her future husband would think of her creative approach to the problem of remaining a virgin in the face of temptation. Frankly, I do not think her plan will even work out, not by a long shot.[3]

---

[3] It depresses me to write it, but her plan did indeed work out well. She got married to a well-off older guy soon after graduating from university. A few years later she divorced him and, in her own words, "got the bigger house and a lot more!" She did not have kids with him. If that was her plan I tip my hat. Well played, slut!

"How do you like my cock?"

I am at Berghain again. It is a great choice for a Friday night because it is such a break from normal life, particularly now that I kind of work. Interning is a pretty bad deal. I deliver work that is better than what many of my colleagues do, and for a fraction of the cost because I am getting paid peanuts. In return I now have a female office mate who is trying to get me kicked out. She spent two weeks trying to summarize the annual report of a large client company but apparently did not pay attention in middle school. Eventually she got frustrated with the numbers, got up and dumped her pile on my desk, telling me to "figure it out!" I was done after a few hours. Now all the ugly women in the office hate me while the two hot ones are still flirting with me. All in all, this place is quite a shit show, so I am not sure whether I should not just quit. Either option is unsatisfactory. My estimation is that I will spend another year or so banging chicks and then I will work on somehow getting my life on track.

I do not have to wear a suit to work and people look at you funny if you dare to. Still, I felt like it today. As I spent a few hours hanging out with colleagues after work — never again! — I really need to change the air. First I head home and take a nap. I wake up at around midnight and put on the same suit again but with cheaper shoes. I mess up my hair, leave two buttons of the dress shirt open, and wear my tie with a badly made four-in-hand knot. Then I loosen it. Now I look as if I have just fucked my secretary. My hair is a mess, my shirt not fully buttoned up, and my tie looks like a noose. I do not think I would get into Berghain dressed properly but this should work. In any case, if they do not let me in I will just fix my appearance and go to some mainstream club instead.

I show up at 1 a.m., which is a bit early, but I really do not want to risk queuing for an hour or so only to be sent away. My outfit is a bit risky, so I want to minimize the potential downside of the bet I made. The two bouncers look at me, then at each other. They let me step sideways to size me up. I think that they are about to tell me to fuck off. Yet, they let me in. Tonight I am clearly a borderline case for this club. Anyway, I am inside and walk around. On Friday the main dance floor is normally not open and that is the case tonight as well. I head straight to Panoramabar on the second floor and ask some tatted up slut of a barkeeper for a glass of tap water. A few people are dancing but it feels quite mellow. The place is slowly filling up.

I observe the environment. A group of three, two girls and a guy, show up next to me. One of the girls looks at me. My eyes are drawn toward her sizable rack. Sadly, the same is true for her thighs and arms. I do not bang fatties, even if they have huge tits. Also, this is not a good sign for this club. I am used to a more selective door policy. Well, they let me in and I am wearing a suit, so that means quite something. I talk to her group for a bit, just to pass some time. They are tourists and they are very excited when I tell them that I, "like really," live in Berlin. They tell me that they have been meeting a lot of tourists and not many authentic people, as they called them. I moved to Berlin myself, so I am not nearly as authentic as all those young men and women who were raised by single mothers on welfare and sent to piss-poor state schools. I do not have any tattoos, nor do I drink or do drugs. In terms of being authentic for Berlin standards, I am clearly not.

I dance for a bit. When I look up a girl makes eye contact and does dance moves from Pulp Fiction. That might be the only association she has with guys in a suit.

"Are you fucking high?", I shout at her. (The music is really loud.)

I do not understand what she says in response because the techno beats completely drown her out. She probably did not understand me either. Anyway, she walks off to her group of friends and grinds into one of the guys in there. I head back to the bar. Several minutes later she is standing next to me.

"Oh, hello there!", I say.

She smiles and says, "I think you're cool!"

"Thanks!"

I put a hand on her waist. She puts one hand on my abs and rubs them. I cup her face. We make intense eye contact. I brush over her luscious lips with my thumb, which she buries in her mouth to suck on. I pull it out of her mouth and go for the kiss, but she is not having any of it.

"So, what brings you here?", I ask.

"I'm traveling around with my boyfriend."

"Your boyfriend?"

"Yeah. He is touring and I just came down from Stockholm to meet up with him."

"What does he do?"

"Oh, he fights in the UFC."

She mentions his name to impress me. I have not heard of him, which does not mean anything. I am not sure if she is kidding or not. That guy could be her boyfriend or someone who just fucks her. It could also be completely made up. However, I am very sure that I do not want to find this out.

"Is your boyfriend in the venue?"

"No, he is not. He'll arrive tomorrow afternoon."

"Okay. Nice meeting you. Have a great night!", I say and give her a quick hug.

I may be bold, but I am not stupid. I meet plenty of women who are overeager to cheat on their boyfriend. If you are playing that kind of game it is better if they do not mention their boyfriend at all or if he is some spineless simp who would not even have the energy to fight you. What you do not want to bother with are women with boyfriends who are trouble, like that UFC fighter who shall not be named.

I sit down for a bit, close my eyes and drift off. When I open my eyes again I notice that a cute girl together with a bunch of other people is sitting next to me. I playfully nudge her with my elbow. She looks at me expectantly.

"I'm sorry, am I sitting on your jacket?", she asks.

"I don't know. I don't care. I just wanted to say hi, so: hi!"

"Hi!"

"I think you're pretty cool. How about we go on a little adventure?"

She giggles. "What do you mean?"

"Give me your hand!"

I extend my hand to her. After some hesitation she takes it. We get up. I walk off with her. The club is now quite busy, so we disappear in the crowd. Her friends probably did not even notice that she is gone. We walk down the hallway that leads to a smaller bar and unisex toilets. She stops. I stop. Then I take her by her waist and lift her up.

"Wow, you're really strong."

"I'm not in the mood to talk."

I push her against the wall. She wraps her arms and legs around me in response. We are making out wildly. After a few moments she turns her head away.

"This is crazy! What is this? Who are you?"

Apparently it is completely out of her reality that a guy acts as quickly as I do.

"At least tell me your name," she says.

"I'm Aaron."

She smiles. We make out again.

"Don't you want to know my name?"

"There is a higher chance I remember it if you tell me afterward."

"I'm not sure I understand."

I grab her pussy.

"I'm sure you do," I say.

She opens her lips ever-so-slightly and moans. I take her hand and head down the stairs with her. Now we are in front of the coat check.

"Um, where exactly are we going?"

"We're going back to my place."

She looks at me.

"This is kind of you," she says and blushes.

I smile.

"Really, I'd love to come with you, but this is too soon. I'm here with one of my flatmates and a girlfriend of mine. I can't leave her with him. I can't be that rude."

"Okay. How do you suggest we handle this?"

"How about you party with us for the rest of the night, and afterward, we, you know ...."

I nod.

"I'm Vee, by the way."

We shake hands.

"I think we rushed things a little bit. Let's do this properly," she says and smiles.

You may now ask why I did not bang her in the venue. Well, do this often enough and you get a good feel for which girl is up for it and which ones prefer proper furniture for sex. This one is probably not the kind of girl who likes to squat down in front of you on the dirty floor of a bathroom stall. I am a bit conflicted. She is pretty good-looking but not a stunner. Then again, I do not have a good alternative right now, so I stick with her for the time being.

After a few minutes her friends start to bore me. We are making lame conversation and the prospect of hanging out with them for a few hours, hoping to get laid at the end, is not that enticing. Another girl in her group, though, is quite foxy. She is also pretty forward. I do not know what is going on between FOXY and VEE. It could well be that FOXY believes she can tease me relentlessly because I will not make a move anyway. Some women are like that. She smiles at me, turns around and shakes her ass in front of me. I grab her by the waist and pull her in. VEE is not happy about this.

FOXY is grinding into me. My pants are quite thin. I am wearing a suit after all. She is wearing a short skirt. This little slut now gyrates her ass against my dick. She is doing some damn fine precision work. I reach inside my pants to make sure my cock is pointing upward and is centered. Foxy presses her ass hard against my cock, moving it up and down rhythmically. Is she trying to make me jizz in my pants? In any case, Vee is really pissed off and walks off. I turn Foxy around, grab her neck and want to make out with her.

"No!", she objects and adds, "I need to talk to my friend first. I think she is upset."

Foxy is quite a cocktease. Now I certainly will not get to fuck Vee and my chances to get with Foxy are slim as well. Consequently, I walk off. Because that chick really made me horny I am now very eager to get laid.

Some buzzed girl throws her arms around me and says, "You are so fucking cool! What's your name?"

"How about we fuck first?"

"You didn't say what I think you said, did you?"

I grab her firmly by the neck. We make intense eye contact. I go for the make out. She aggressively shoves her tongue down my throat. Before I can get anywhere with her half a dozen girls show up and drag her off. They form a circle around her to prevent her from doing something she might enjoy.

As I walk around someone is pinching my ass. I turn around and look straight into the face of the supposed culprit.

"Don't look at me. He did it!", she says, pointing at her gay-looking friend.

"No, I didn't do it," he stammers.

After another pinch I turn around and face that girl again. Let's call her PINCHER. I put my hand on her lower back and pull her in.

"You're really forward!", I say.

"No, I think you are *really* forward."

"I can tell that you like it", I say as I firmly grab her tight ass.

"Yes, I do."

We make out. I better capitalize on this. FOXY managed to get me very horny and I want to get some action now. I take PINCHER by the hand and drag her off. I mean, I try. She resists quite strongly for a few seconds. I turn around and say, "Come now!", as I keep pulling. This does the trick. She follows me willingly.

First I check those semi-open boxes next to the dance floor at Panoramabar. They are all occupied. It is not as if people are fucking out in the open. Some people take a nap, others sit there and cuddle, some sit around and share drinks. It is all pretty tame. Then I take PINCHER to the unisex bathroom. Like a professional, obviously, I calmly check one door after another until I find a vacant stall after five or six tries.

I usher PINCHER in, follow, and lock the door behind me. We make out. Meanwhile, I put her hands on my upper body. Moments later I unzip my pants and pull my dick out. I break the make out, put one of her hands on my dick and gesture with my head that she should go down on me. She squats down right away and takes my dick in her mouth. We are about three minutes into the interaction. I am not sure this can be done much quicker. Plenty of times I have made out with girls right away. Those instant make outs are nothing special at all for me anymore. Before I started experimenting with blowjobs and sex in the venue I sometimes went for a handjob on the dance floor or in a dark corner. Those can be had within one or two minutes, too, if you find the right girl. Now I have apparently graduated to instant blowjobs.

She is sucking eagerly on my dick. I'm getting harder and harder. The moment I get really hard she starts deep-throating. I grab her by the hair on the back on her head and pull her back. She is now sucking just on the tip of my cock.

"How do you like my cock?", I ask her.

She winks. I move her head back and forth, ramming my cock down her throat. She is accompanying this with, "Mmm."

Then, all of a sudden, she puts both hands on my thighs and stops. I back off. Before I can say anything she laments loudly, "Shit, I left my handbag behind." She jumps up.

"Quick, we have to go! We have to go!", she urges me.

Before I can put my dick away she has already opened the door. We are rushing back to her friend. Her friend is gone. Her handbag is not. It is on the floor, right next to the Panoramabar counter. It is a good thing that Berghain is a pretty dark club. Otherwise someone could easily have taken her handbag. It looks like a pretty expensive one, too.

"I'm so glad nobody took it," she says and adds, "Now let me calm down. This was a bit too exciting for me."

We first sit down, chit-chatting. She wants to buy me a drink but because I do not drink she gets me a glass of water.

"How about we dance for a bit," she suggests.

"Sure."

"But please behave yourself!"

That is easier said than done.

"Hold on to your handbag," I say.

She laughs. Minutes later we are back in a bathroom stall. I blow a load quickly; she swallows with visible delight. Yes, there are no details because there will be plenty of juicy details later and I do not want to tire you out.

We head back to the dance floor. Now her friend joins us. We all sit down by the windows, enjoying the music and making some small talk. PINCHER is cuddling up to me. She is like a puppy. Time just flies.

"I don't know what your plan is, but I want to party until they kick us out," she says.

"When do they close?"

"At around noon."

There is no way I am going to stick around for that long. Right now it is around 7 or 8 a.m., which I consider very late. It is good that I took a long nap before going out. It has also been about two hours since I have blown a load. I am getting horny again.

"I have to go to the toilet. Wait here, I'll be back in five minutes," she says.

"I'll come with you."

We are entering the unisex bathroom. The first stall is unoccupied. She turns around and says, "Give me two minutes."

She enters the stall on her own and locks the door behind her. After a little while the door unlocks and she opens it. I step toward her, raise my hand to the level of her chest and nonchalantly gesture that she should go back inside.

Then things get a little bit crazy. She slips out of her thin dress, rolls it up and stuffs it into her handbag, which she puts down in a corner. She is squatting down in front of me, grabbing my dick and stroking it. Soon afterward my dick is in her mouth again. Her blowjob skills are quite phenomenal this time. It seems she held back before. I do not want to blow another load in her mouth. At least not yet. Besides, I should appreciate that she undressed for me. She looks really slutty, with her high leather boots and just her panties on.

I gesture her to get up. Meanwhile, I pull a condom out of my jacket, tear it open and put it on. She is spitting on my dick and stroking it. Then she turns around, still holding my cock, bends forward, and puts it in. I grab her by the waist and push hard.

"Aaaahhhhh," she moans.

She is pressing against the wall with both hands and pushing back really hard, synchronized with each of my hard thrusts. I have to say that I am very impressed by how great a fuck she is. Partly it is surely due to her height. Her pussy is exactly where my cock wants it to be. Then there is the visual aspect. I see her long mane flying around — I bet she has hair extensions — and apart from that, she is essentially naked. The only piece of clothing she wears is her panties, which have given way for my cock. Oh, and those slutty boots!

Judging from how she acts I bet she has done this more

than a few times before. For a moment or two I even wonder whether she is merely going through a routine, so smooth did it go from opening the door to the bathroom stall to fucking her. She is bending over, pushing hard into the wall, and giving me not just a pushback but on top she also makes a slight rolling motion with her pelvis which feels amazing.

I am pounding away.

"Take it!", I shout.

"I'm all yours. Aaahhh! Fuck me! Aaaahhhhh!"

"I'm fucking you, slut!"

"I'm your slut. Aaahhhhhhhh! Give it to me harder!"

"How's that? Huh, how's that?"

I am spouting literature Nobel prize worthy lines here.

"Aaaahhhhh! Fuck me with your big cock! Aaaahhhhh!"

I am pounding her as hard and as fast as I can. I want to blow a load in her. She does not seem to like that idea as she breaks the rhythm and somehow bumps me off. Did she really sense that I was about to come or did she deduce this from me fucking her faster and faster? I wonder what is going on.

She turns around, squats down, pulls the condom off my cock, and proceeds with giving me the most amazing blowjob ever. After she pulled the condom off, my cock got soft for a bit, but she quickly fixes that. Her first move is to take it in all the way. She makes gentle sucking motions while staring at me with her eyes wide open. My cock is getting bigger and bigger. Once I am almost fully erect she transitions into deep-throating with an interesting sequence: first she takes my dick in all the way. When pulling back she presses her tongue against my shaft from below, followed by touching the frenulum of my cock with the tip of her tongue. Then she sucks on the tip of my cock really hard, and so on. All of this is accompanied by a lot of moaning and slurping that show how much she enjoys sucking my dick. There is not a single dull moment in that blowjob. Every movement is one of a true master of this art. I am steadily getting more and more aroused.

Now she is increasing the speed. She is also increasing the pressure of her tongue and sucking harder as well. I am getting close. I want to come. Moments later I start blowing a load. Right after blowing the first part of my load she pulls my dick out and waves it in front of her face. With a big smile she is giving herself a facial. I am done. This was great!

"Oh, Aaron!", she says.

Then she sucks on the tip of my cock again until I have to gesture that she should stop because I am getting too sensitive. Meanwhile, my cum is running down her face. I hand her a handkerchief, which she uses to clean her face. Then she licks my entire dick up and down a few times, pretending to clean it. In reality she is showing her great admiration for my big cock.

We are done.

"Now I really need to clean my face. I hope I don't look too bad," she says and laughs. There are no mirrors in the bathrooms at Berghain but she has a pocket mirror in her handbag, which she uses to check that she looks like a proper lady again. Then she puts on her dress again.

We are leaving the bathroom stall. She turns around and smiles at me.

"How about you buy me a drink now?", she asks with a sexy smile.

"I'd love to, but I'm broke."

"Okay. It's on me then."

We are back at Panoramabar. She is getting us drinks. I have some orange juice; her choice is orange juice with vodka. Then we sit down again, cuddling, talking, kissing. All boundaries are gone now. She unbuttons my shirt, then licks, bites, and sucks my nipples. She bites my neck and scratches my back. A little later she takes my shirt halfway off and licks my arm and she keeps going: she licks my nipples with the tip of her tongue and uses her whole tongue moments later to lick my chest, shoulder, and arms. Finally, she puts my index finger in her mouth and sucks on it. We are out in the open but she does not care. I do not care anyway.

While she is devouring me some other girl walks over, stops and stares at me. She is eyeball-fucking me. My chick takes my index finger out of her mouth and turns around to lean into me. Now she sees that other girl who has been staring at me. They exchange some unfriendly glances. That poor girl seems embarrassed by that and scuttles off.

"Do you really want to stay until noon?", I ask her.

"Yes, I do."

"That's too bad. I'm getting quite sleepy and would rather sleep in my bed. I think I'm heading off now."

"You can go home and rest. You have every right to be exhausted," she says, while giving me a big smile.

She buttons up my shirt and pretends to fix my hair. We exchange one last firm hug. Then I am off. I intermittently fall asleep on public transport and almost miss my stop. I think I will stay in this Saturday.

Surprise Visit

Because my Friday night was pretty extreme — I only came back home at around 9.30 or 10.00 a.m. — I stayed in on Saturday to recover. The problem is that if I go to bed at that time my sleeping schedule will be completely ruined. Instead, I try staying awake. I have breakfast, shower, and then watch a few classic James Bond movies. I crash at around 3 p.m., which is not so bad, and wake up around 16 hours later, on Sunday morning. This is a fine outcome because this means that I should be able to get up without much of a problem on Monday morning. I do not feel like getting up, so I snooze until around noon.

My phone vibrates. A text message has arrived.

"Hey! I'm in Berlin for the wknd. Leaving 2nite. Coffee? xxx"

What kind of gibberish is that? I have no idea who this is anyway because I purge my phone of text messages and phone numbers of the women I meet in regular intervals. This also helps me avoid any drama because once I wipe a girl's contact data from my phone and on social media I cannot contact them anymore and because women are generally passive this arrangement leads to great peace of mind. Drama normally comes once you meet them repeatedly.

I still have a good 10 hours to kill before I can go back to bed and I have nothing planned. I kind of feel like banging one of my fuck buddies, but I am also curious who just texted me. I do not exchange phone numbers with unattractive women, so I do not think this can end badly. I text back, "Hey! Great to hear from you! Meet me at Schoenhauser Allee outside Coffee Balzac at 2 p.m."

Almost immediately I get the response: "Great! CU there xox!!"

There is also the risk that some disgruntled simp shows up whose girlfriend or wife I have fucked, ready to take me on. The meeting point is a busy place, so I have a hard time imagining how this would play out. I take care of things and eventually saunter from my apartment down to that coffee shop. There I sit down on one of the benches, wondering who will show up.

It is slightly past 2 p.m. and no girl seems to be arriving for me. Well, girls are hardly ever on time, so I stick around for a few more minutes. I get a text, "Sry, still on the way. cu in 5." Oh well, I may as well wait this one out.

Then some girl squeaks and runs toward me.

"Aaron, Aaron!", she shouts and rushes toward me with her arms stretched out. I get up. She wraps her arms around me.

"Aaron, Aaron, it's so good to see you again! How have you been?"

"Great. What about you?"

Now you may want to know who that girl is. It is one I am indeed happy to see again. It is Orgasm Girl from the opening chapter of this book. I cannot say that I am not getting a boner as she hugs me, pressing her tits firmly against my chest.

"How much time do we have?", I ask.

"Two hours or so. I have to meet someone at 4 p.m."

We clearly do not have time for coffee. I take her hand and walk in the direction of my apartment.

"There is a great place I'd like to take you to," I say.

She is giddy in anticipation. On the way she tells me that she has decided to study in Heidelberg but that she loves Berlin. I also get to hear the most inane bullshit about people I have not even met. She just keeps babbling on.

After a few minutes with no cafe in sight she gets a bit skeptical.

"Wait, where exactly are we going?", she asks.

I do not answer. Instead, I shove her against the nearest wall and ram my tongue into her mouth. She goes along with it.

"Just like I remember you!", she gushes.

We continue walking. A few minutes later her curiosity gets the upper hand again.

"You didn't tell me where we are going. Where are we going, Aaron?"

"I have some stuff at my place to take care of."

"I didn't expect this but, okay, I guess."

Shortly afterward we are in my apartment building. In the hallway to my apartment I pull her in, put one hand on her ass, and with the other I grab her head. We are making out.

"I'm not sure I ...," she says.

"I know."

We are in my apartment. I hear two of my flatmates talking in our kitchen.

"The kitchen is busy. We have to hang out in my room then," I say.

I open the door to my room and usher her in.

"How about you take your shoes off," I reprimand her.

"Oh, sorry!"

"While you're at it ...," I say and start undressing her.

We are undressing each other. Unlike back then in the club we now have plenty of space, so I first lift her up and throw her onto my bed. I am on top of her. I dangle my cock in front of her face and she quickly grabs it with her mouth. I am on my knees. She looks up to me, worshipping my cock. Now I grab her head with both hands and vehemently yank it back and forth as I ram my cock down her throat.

"Mmm! Mmmm!," she comments.

I pull my dick out and position myself for sixty-nine. She is already working on my dick. I think this through once more and conclude that I do not want to go down on her. She gets my finger instead.

"Aaaahh! Aaaahhh!," she moans.

That is enough foreplay. I grab a condom while jerking my cock and hold the condom in front of her face.

"Do you want to help me out here?," I ask.

She eagerly tears the wrapper open, deep-throats me for a few long and very enjoyable moments and afterward puts the condom on my cock.

"Turn around!", I order her.

She does what I tell her. I get behind her, shove my hard cock into her pussy, and ram her hard.

"Aaahh! Aaaahhh! Aaaaahhhh!," she moans as I am pounding her.

She has her ass in the air and rests her head on my bed. With her arms she reaches around and pulls her ass apart. I can help her out with that. I play with her asshole and with one elegant movement I grab the bottle of lube on my desk and flick it open. I lube her up and to top it off I fuck her in the ass as well.

"Aaaaaaahhh! Aaaaaaaaaaahhhhh!"

I wonder what my neighbors think of this but in the end I do not really care. I just want to blow a load, so I pull out, throw her on her back, and pull the condom off. I put my dick in her mouth. She is sucking me. Then she is sucking only the tip of it, hard, while I'm jerking myself. I am about to come. To spice up my boring weekend I yank my dick out of her mouth and blow a load all over her face.

Her "Ewww!" goes very nicely with my, "Mmmmaah!"

After I am done she properly cleans my cock with her tongue.

"That was naughty," she diagnoses.

"That was great," I say and add, "clean yourself up and I'll make you come as well."

"I wonder how bad I look."

"No worries. You only have to walk past my flatmates. The bathroom is at the other end of the apartment."

"That's not funny."

She rummages through her handbag and pulls out a pocket mirror. She flips it open, looks at herself in the mirror — and throws it at me. I laugh.

"That's not funny, asshole!"

"Get a grip. Here, take this hankie and wipe my cum off your face. I have three female flatmates and they keep their beauty products in the bathroom. Just take whatever you need to make yourself look presentable." (What can I say, I am a generous person.)

"That's not the issue. I also have some of your cum in my hair!", she protests.

"I thought that was the point," I argue and cannot stop laughing.

She scowls at me.

"Hey, come here!", I say.

I give her a hug and pat her back, followed by a slap on her ass. She calms down.

"Sorry, I didn't mean to get mad at you. What you've done with me was really hot."

She is wiping her face. I am not sure that her totally smeared makeup looks better than my cum.

"You know what, we'll get you to look prim and proper again. Put your dress on and then put this on your head!", I say as I hand her a dry towel.

After covering her head and face with my towel I lead her to the bathroom. My flatmates look a bit befuddled, but my chick is fine. It is the same principle that works with toddlers: if you cover their eyes they believe the world no longer exists.

In the bathroom we take a shower together. I also make her suck my dick for a bit, just because I can. Of course I do not yet have the energy to blow another load. The dried cum she gets out with a comb. Then, to be on the safe side, she washes and blow-dries her hair. Afterward she fixes her makeup. After what feels like an eternity she is finally done. We head back to my room.

She walks into my room in front of me. I grab her from behind in a surprise attack and start working on her clitoris. A little later I lift her up and sit her down on my desk. I stretch her out. She is lying down. I have one hand on her clit, the other is in her pussy, massaging her G-spot. I should have become a gynecologist, specializing in attractive teenage girls. Anyway, I pull my pants down and put my dick in her mouth, which she treats well with her tongue. As I think that we are pressed for time I pull my dick out of her mouth again and fully focus on getting her off. I start by giving her a clitoral orgasm. After that is done I give her a few minutes to cool off before I continue with her G-spot. She comes once more.

"Again?", I ask.

"I'm not sure I can again that soon. We're not in a club."

"We'll just see," I say and start over, hammering her G-spot. Minutes later she comes again.

"Now it's your turn again," I tell her.

She smiles.

"Kneel before me!", I command her.

She does that. Then she pulls my pants down and takes my dick into her mouth and gets to work. After a few good thrusts, she stops and pulls my dick out of her mouth again.

"If you give me another facial, I'll kill you!", she says.

I chuckle.

She gets back to work and sucks me really well, and very eagerly. This is probably her insurance that I am not blowing a load all over her face again, and so it was.

I end up shooting a load down her throat, accompanied by one "Mmm!" after another.

"It's really been fun catching up with you, Aaron!", she says and winks.

"I think so, too. Oh, don't you have to head off soon?"

"Shit, that's right. Well, I'll just be late then. Um, do you have something to drink at home, coffee maybe?"

"Sure."

We walk into the kitchen while she texts someone on the phone. My flatmates say hi, awkwardly, and I prepare coffee with a French press.

"Thanks! I just wanted to have a different taste in my mouth," she says as I hand her a cup of coffee. This is accompanied by a mischievous smile. One of my female flatmates throws a vile look at her as she hears that.

We hang out in my room some more. At around 5 p.m., she is getting ready to leave the apartment. She turns toward me and asks, "I don't think I'll find my way back. Would you mind accompanying me to Schön-hauser Allee?"

I walk her back. On the way she tells me that she is in Berlin with her boyfriend, whom she has told to spend some time on his own. I chuckle and wonder if there are only sluts left on this planet or if those women are all I am ever going to meet.

We arrive at Schönhauser Allee. It is a busy station as well as a popular meeting point late in the afternoon. There are plenty of shady characters around. I see drug dealers, beggars, and punks with shaggy dogs. Yet, this is one of the more affluent districts of this city. Berlin is fucked.

"I told my boyfriend to meet me at Schönhauser Allee, but I don't really feel safe around here. Um, could you please wait here with me?"

"You're kidding, right?"

"I'm not. Just look around! Look at these people!"

"OK. But what are you going to tell your boyfriend about who I am?"

"You're just some acquaintance. I told him you're one of my gay friends so he doesn't needlessly worry."

"Me, gay? Thanks!"

"Hey! You totally look like a faggot. It's a compliment, so cheer up, stud!"

I smirk. She wraps one arm around me. With her free hand she grabs my junk and squeezes it.

"I love your cock," she whispers in my ear.

"How about we take your boyfriend into consideration?"

"Thankfully there's a big crowd here."

After a while she lets go. She looks around and eventually she spots her boyfriend in the crowd. She probably let him wait for an hour. He looks like your typical beta provider simp who got ignored by women until he got a decently well-paying job.

"This is my gay friend Aaron," she says while pointing at me. Moments later he gets a peck on his lips. If only he knew. I shudder.

We shake hands.

"Nice to meet you!", I say.

"Same."

"I have to go. Nice meeting you. Have a safe trip home, and good luck!", I say.

I walk back home and I am appalled, thinking of the morals of our times. You can now of course say that if guys like me were not around, those women would not cheat on their boyfriends, but I do not think that is necessarily true. They would simply fuck someone else instead. It better be me.

No Kissing Allowed

I recently listened to an interview with the aged music star Gene Simmons on National Public Radio. It was quite obvious that he wanted to provoke the female interviewer. He just did not give a fuck. One of his statements was that women wanted to "perform sexual favors" on him as an expression of their appreciation. Your average Joe does not know what this is like, but when I heard this it struck a chord with me as it is the case that some women are very eager to sexually please me. This is most obvious when they spread their legs for me and only want me to fuck them or when they suck me off in a bathroom stall and do not expect anything in return. In those instances the mere validation of having sexually served a guy like me is apparently enough for them.

I have a particularly fitting story to tell you on that note. It is Friday and I am in the mood for checking out a different venue than the same few places I frequent over and over, like Berghain and Watergate for techno music or Magnet Club and Bang Bang Club for indie rock. Thus, I head to Tresor, which is one of the longest-running techno clubs in Berlin. I was there once before, soon after I had moved to Berlin for the first time but did not like it that much. However, that was before I had figured out how to turn clubs into a never-ending stream of pussy.

I should have known better. Among my friends and acquaintances who like going to techno clubs there is not a single one who has been to Tresor in the last few years. When I asked around a few people even wanted to know whether I am sure that this club is still in operation. That did not put an end to my curiosity. I thought that if Tresor manages to survive in a location somewhat off the beaten path in Berlin it cannot be that bad. So, I walk in after queueing for a bit and I am quite impressed. The architecture is captivating and the music quite original. I am used to only minimal techno being played in clubs, but here they are putting on electronic music with jazz influences. It is pretty great.

Okay, the venue is nice and the music is great. Let's get laid! I systematically prowl the venue and mostly bump into men. They look a bit older than the usual party crowd. I look young for my age. I am close to 30 and quite old for partying it up and banging sluts in bathroom stalls, so I conclude that I may just have happened to be in a club catering to people my age. Unfortunately, the women are also a bit older. The look of a woman around 30, in particular a used up Western one, does not cause a rush of blood to my cock like it is the case with hot, young sluts. If I had no other choice I could consider hitting on one or two of the women in here but they just are not appealing enough. I briefly speak to probably the most attractive woman in the venue. She tells me that she is here with a bunch of colleagues and business acquaintances. They are celebrating the successful completion of a consulting project. Really, this is not quite the crowd I am used to. It is time to leave.

I head outside, pondering what to do. After this disaster I do not want to risk walking into another venue and not getting anything in return. Thus, it has to be a reasonably safe bet. Besides, it is not as if I am particularly flush with money. I spend ten to fifteen Euros on cover charge at those clubs, but that is enough to feed me for at least two days. Going to comparatively expensive places two days in a row, let alone in one night, is not what I would call great value for money. (Maybe it is time I look for a proper job.) Then I think that I am almost guaranteed to get some action at Berghain, so I head there straight away.

I arrive at around 2:30 a.m. The queue is not even that

bad. Within twenty minutes I am inside. Because the main dance floor does not tempt me I head upstairs to Panoramabar instead. I arrive at just the right moment as the crowd is already captivated by the beat of the music. It is not nearly as creative as what I just listened to at Tresor, but it does the trick. After walking around the venue and checking out tonight's menu it is time to get to work. The offering is quite delicious tonight! The first woman who catches my attention is SKULL. She is about my height. I am freaking out a little bit, but feel better after noticing that she is wearing obscenely high heels. Overall, she looks spectacular! Her brunette hair extends down to her lower back, she is slender and toned and she has a very symmetrical face with big eyes and high cheekbones. I do not want to bullshit you that she is supermodel caliber — her tits are way too big for that — but she is very good-looking by any standard.

On her tight black top there is a big print of a skull. Its eye sockets encircle her nipples, which are quite visible now that they are stiff. That is a creative as well as provocative outfit. Her super-tight black jeans and heels further complement it. I calmly walk toward her on the dance floor. She pretends to not notice me, but steps on my foot. I take her hand and pull her in. We dance for a little bit. I pull all the stops. First I lift her up and quickly dip her. She shrieks and throws her arms around me.

"You're insane!", she says.

"I know."

I turn her around, grab her pussy and pull her in so that she can grind that marvelous ass against my dick. She is gyrating it like a pro. We are having a lot of fun. Unbeknownst to me we would only have a few minutes together because some guy shows up.

"This is my big brother!", she says and introduces us.

They briefly talk to each other. Then SKULL turns back to me.

"He says he really has to go to an industry party now; he is a TV director. I promised I'd drive him, so I unfortunately have to go now."

I can tell that she is really into me and, yes, I find her extremely attractive as well. As a bit of foreshadowing I let you know that she has a side-gig as a glamour model, mostly doing lingerie. Pictures of her appeared in magazines. She also did leg-modeling for a campaign for a manufacturer of stockings, which ended up on posters all over Germany and possibly abroad, too. Anyway, hers is a story for another chapter.

"I think we should stay in touch. How about you give me your phone number!", I say.

"Yeah, of course!"

She keys it into my phone.

"And now call me so I have your number, too!"

She takes both my hands. You can tell that she is very enthusiastic.

"I'm sorry that I have to go. I can tell that you're really fun."

"Yeah, I think you're really fun too. Listen, I'm busy on Monday. What are your plans for Tuesday evening?"

She looks at me with big eyes. Then she smiles and says, "Meeting you again — that's my plan for Tuesday evening!"

She plants a big kiss on my cheek, and off she is. I probably have lipstick on my face now. I cannot check it myself as I do not have a mirror in my pocket and the bathrooms are likewise without mirrors. Thus, I grab the first girl and ask her, "Do I have lipstick on my face?"

"Yeah, you do, asshole. Gosh, you guys really don't give a fuck anymore."

She is furrowing her eyebrows.

"Hey, easy! It was just a question."

"Get away from me! I probably would have liked you, but not if you're coming on to me like that."

Okay. I walk off. I was not even hitting on her and had no intention of doing so to begin with.

I head to the unisex toilets to make myself look presentable. As I walk in a pretty cute girl is leaving one of the stalls. I abort my plan and instead turn around and walk after her. She is in quite a hurry. I grab her hand. She is taking it away instinctively, but at the same time she is checking me out. She stops, turns around, and smiles coyly. I take one of her wrists, then the other, and finally I hold both wrists with one hand. She is frozen in eager anticipation. Her eyes are gleaming, her lips are parted. I gently push her against the wall, followed by pressing her wrists against the wall as well, over her head.

"You can't just walk off like that," I say.

She keeps looking at me and presses her loins against mine. Yet, she tries to wrestle her hands free. I grant her partial freedom. She is pressing her loins harder against me, but at the same time she pretends to want to push me away.

I laugh.

"I guess I'm not very convincing," she says.

"No, you're not."

I lift her up and carry her deeper into the hallway. My goal is one of those semi-open enclosures next to the dance floor at Panoramabar.

"Where are you taking me?", she says while she is playing with my hair with one hand and rubbing my back with the other.

"I haven't decided yet."

I arrive at my destination and put her down. She immediately hugs me, intensively.

"It's not that I don't like you. I do. But I'm here with friends of mine. If I'm gone for too long, they'll look for me. Also, I don't want any rumors to spread at school, so I have to go back to them."

She hugs me again.

"Okay. I'll probably hunt you down later."

"What, don't you want my number?"

"Nah, I'll find you."

"Oh."

She looks disappointed and walks off.

I dance on my own for a bit and bop my head to the music. It is about time some other chick catches my attention, but it has been slim pickings for a while. Then a woman who looks like a heavy partier walks past. She is dressed in white from head to heels. I would say she is in her mid-twenties. Judging by the jaded look on her face and her tattoos she could as well be only eighteen or nineteen. A steady diet of booze, coke, and cock really does age women. Add sleep deprivation and poor nutrition to it and you end up with the kind of woman you want to approach if you just want to get laid. Anyway, she is making her way through the crowd. She looks at me, then she looks away and tries walking past me. I block her path, put my hand on her lower back and pull her in.

"Hello there!", I say with a sleazy smile.

She looks at me but does not show much enthusiasm.

"No worries, I can deal with stuck-up chicks," I say.

She laughs.

"No, it's not that. I've been looking for someone, a friend, not for some dude to hook up with."

"You're not?"

"Um, not right now at least."

"Let's explore that line of thought somewhere else," I say and take her hand. I drag her off but then I feel some resistance.

"Wait, wait!", she shrieks.

Some gay-looking dude is holding her back. Oh, there are two of them.

"These are my friends!", she tells me.

"Sorry, jerk-off, but that guy here is her boyfriend," he says. Even in the loud atmosphere of a club his voice comes across as quite nasal.

"Sure, dickwad. I can tell without looking that both of you prefer cock," I retort.

We hold eye contact. He does not say a word. Neither am I. Then he burst out laughing and puts his arm around me. I ignore that he is squeezing my neck and shoulders and rub his lower back for a bit, not because I have bisexual tendencies, which I do not have, but because that is an easy way to show that you are cool with being around gay guys. You certainly do not want some faggot to torpedo your pickup because he does not like you.

"You're alright, mate, you're alright!", he says.

All three of us laugh.

"What's so funny?", the chick asks. We both shrug our shoulders. Then we laugh some more.

The second gay dude now comes closer and high fives me.

"I think you're a cool dude," he says.

"Thanks, man."

"Those shoes you're wearing…. What brand is that and where did you get them from?"

"These? These are Ed Hardy sneakers."

I do not even like them that much, but they fit well and I got them for cheap at some designer outlet store the other week.

"They look comfortable."

"They are."

His attempts at putting me down are not working. I have been talking for far too long to those gay dudes now, so I grab that girl's wrist and pull her in.

"About time," she says as she wraps her arms around me.

"Are you French by any chance?"

I get this a lot. I do not reply but instead look into her eyes, which she reciprocates. We stare into each other's eyes. We are close to making out, but the gay dude I was just talking to is having none of it.

"You know what, you'd have to only pay something like ten euros for that in Poland," he says.

"Probably. But it's not the same because I quite enjoy the hunt."

He bursts out laughing.

"What's up with you guys?", she interjects.

"You have to hear this: I teased him, telling him that he would only have to pay around ten euros in Poland. Of course, I'm talking about his gaudy Ed Hardy shoes but he thought I was talking about you."

They both laugh.

That gay dude grabs me by the neck, pricks my chest with the other hand and says to her, "This guy is a crazy mofo. Watch out!" I take this as a sign of approval. In any case, I think I have been wasting enough time talking to those dudes, so I take her hand and drag her off. This time they do not interfere. Instead, one of them shouts, "See you later. Have fun!" They did not interfere because they now like me. She follows willingly. We walk past Panoramabar and toward those semi-open booths. We stand in front of the first empty one I see.

She looks at me.

"You are not going to get me into one of those. No way!", she protests.

"Come on!"

"No! It's totally gross."

To be fair, gay men often use those booths for sex and I am not sure how often they get cleaned, if at all. I take her back to the bar, where we sit down on one of the sofas. She is like a changed person now and takes the conversation over. Her eyes are glowing.

"You're picking up a different woman every time you go out, right? I totally know your type," she claims.

"You mean hot guys?"

She slaps my chest. "Shut up! You're so full of yourself!"

Now she is rubbing my chest. Her lips are very close to mine. I can feel her breath.

"Tell me, do you fuck a new girl every week?"

I put her hand on the bulge in my crotch, which she rubs.

"Is this a yes?", she says and laughs.

I put my hand on her hand and make sure that she keeps a good rhythm going. Then I notice that her skin feels very dry.

"Oh, why is your skin so dry?"

She hastily pulls her hand away, hides it behind her back, and looks down to the floor. I look at her expectantly. After a while she looks up and crosses her arms.

"I'll tell you. My skin is dry because of atopic dermatitis. I got an allergic reaction the other day and ended up scratching myself way too much. It's pretty bad."

"Oh," I say as I embrace her.

Making her talk about her skin condition killed the mood. I did not expect that answer at all. My best guess was that she had gotten into a fight with her cat. Oh well, it looks as if this is it. She moves away from me. I move toward her.

"I'm sorry. I did not mean to make you feel uncomfortable," I say.

"I know. It's nothing you could have known, but now I feel ugly and unattractive. I'm really sorry. I think I should get back to my friends."

She quickly spots them, so I accompany her. After a bit of friendly banter I wish them a great night and walk off. The sexual vibe between that girl and me had completely disappeared.

The night is not going particularly great but I still have a few hours left. After a while I spot a woman who is seemingly on her own. It is a good idea to prioritize women who are out on their own because it is generally quite easy to lay them. That is probably the wrong way to put it. Instead, the issue is that they tend to desperately want to get laid and if it is not your turn then it will be someone else's. Still, she might be yours for the taking. I grab her hand and pull her in, to which she responds with a big smile. As this is an excellent sign I just lead her off. There are two porch swings at Berghain and I am curious to see if they are taken. They are both in a room that is quite dark, so you can easily get a blowjob there or even fuck. No, not just me; I have seen people bang on them.

"Where are you taking me?", she giddily says.

"Just wait. It'll be fun."

"Okay."

We are standing in front of one of those porch swings. I

sit down, lean back and gesture her to sit down as well.

"Was this the tackiest thing you could think of?"

"Hey, I didn't have a lot of time."

She laughs and sits down. I put my arm around her and pull her in. Moments later she is sitting on my lap. We lock eye contact. Our heads are moving closer together. I can feel her breath on my lips. Then she snaps out of it and playfully hits me on the chest, "So that's what I get for going to a gay night! All I wanted was to dance and now look at this: You're probably one out of a dozen or so straight guys in this place and you already got your fangs in me."

"Oh, do I?", I say as I squeeze her tight ass.

"Wow, you're really forward."

"You're the one with the i..., I mean the flowery language, so don't complain."

I almost would have said "idiom," but I cannot say that using big words ever helped me much with getting laid. You do not want to intimidate chicks. She laughs and adds, "Yeah, you got a point. By the way, I think the word you were looking for was 'idiom.'"

"I have no idea what you're talking about," I bullshit.

"Whatever," she says softly, while caressing my chest with her fingertips and gazing deeply into my eyes. I go for the kiss. She tries pushing me back and averts her neck, which I nibble at. She laughs.

"No, seriously, I really only wanted to dance tonight. But, but … . Well, screw it!"

She grabs the hair on the back of my head with one hand, the other is under my T-shirt, gently scratching my skin. Meanwhile, she is shoving her tongue down my throat. That is one aggressive chick! Yet, I am not getting a strong sexual vibe from her. No, really, hear me out: She is very mechanical, almost calculating. It is as if she wants to hit a few triggers to arouse me. She is doing this very well, but I do not sense a lot of passion. My best bet is that she has gone through so many cocks that sexual escalation has become nothing but a routine procedure to go through. I have had more than my fair share of women but I do not think I am like that as I do not just go through the motions.

"I can tell that you're a lot of fun, but I think I want to enjoy the music some more," she says.

"Sure. I'll see you around, then."

"No, that's not what I meant. How about we dance together."

We head back to Panoramabar.

My perception is that it would take me a few hours to get her out of the club, if at all. She also seems way too much in control of her sexuality, so sex in some bathroom stall would not happen so easily, except if she wanted it, and if she wanted it she would probably lead me there herself. I would not be surprised if she is an escort or at least a part-time whore. Regular women just do not have as much control over their sex drive as she does. They are also not as sexually aggressive.

On the dance floor she presses her tits firmly against me and wraps her arms around my neck. After some kissing she tells me to wait for her.

"I'll be right back. Just let me take care of something," she says. Then she walks off.

That is as good as any other moment to move on. The interaction with her did feel a bit off and when I am in doubt I listen to my gut feeling. As soon as she turns around to walk off, I notice some other girl staring at me. As I am about to make my way toward her my phone buzzes. It is BYTE! He writes that he is on the way to a club called Golden Gate and invites me to tag along. "I'm already at Berghain. I'll be in touch," I reply. When I look up from my phone that chick I wanted to approach is making out with some dude. She just grabbed him and tongued him down and now she is pushing him away already. I do not quite know how I should interpret this. Maybe he had no clue how to handle her. He could also have been a bad kisser. Anyway, he walks off and she is dancing on her own again. She is also staring at me once more. I slowly walk up to her. She stops moving.

I take her wrist and pull her in. She responds by pressing her lower body against mine, wrapping her arms around my neck, and rhythmically rubbing her crotch against my leg. From what I can tell she only wants attention. I lean in to kiss her, but then I grab her neck and guide her head to my shoulders, which she happily proceeds to suck on. She is pretty hot but as she has just made out with some random guy I do not want to follow up right away. She is turning her attention away from my shoulders to my neck and then my earlobe. I gently push her head back, take her drink and press it against her lips. She is taking a sip.

"Have some more," I say.

She follows my orders.

Now I feel more comfortable making out with her. She is getting into it and claws my ass with her sharp fingernails. As the dance floor is quite dark I take the liberty of reaching into her top and playing with her nipples. Given how small her breasts are, this is not a lot of fun, so I grab her ass in return. She is slender and in excellent shape. A boob job would do wonders for her appearance, though.

Now she turns around, presses her ass against my groin, and flings her hair around manically. She is certainly not following the minimal techno beat of the music.

Instead, she follows the beat of a different drummer. She does not even flinch when I take one of her hands and put it on my crotch. Instead, she rests her left hand on her knee while she is pushing her ass into me, which barely hides that she is fondling my cock. She is just a cock-tease, though. When I turn her around, she flings her arms around the first semi-attractive dude she sees and tries dancing seductively with him. He is freaking out and freezing up. I chuckle and walk off.

Dealing with that woman was a bit of a waste of time, but now I am really horny and eager to get my rocks off. I look around some more on the dance floor, searching for a woman to use as an outlet for my pent-up sexual energy. While slowly making my way through the crowd I notice a short Spanish-looking girl with very nice curves. By that I mean that she has an hourglass figure, a very nice rack and, presumably, a nice ass. (When a woman says she is "curvy" she normally just does not want to say that she is fat, but that is not what the former means.)

She looks at me spellbound. Her lips are parted. I stand right in front of her and she reciprocates by shyly looking down to the floor. I take her hand.

"Look up!", I say.

She looks up and gives me this incredibly sexy smile. I pull her in. Her hands are all over me. Someone really wants it, it seems. Unlike that cold whore from before or the cocktease I just met this girl means business. I hold her close and stare into her eyes. She is getting hornier by the second. It is cute how she stands up on her toes in an attempt to get close to my neck. I pull back. Then I grab her firmly by her waist and look deep into her eyes.

"You're a cruel man," she says.

I do not say anything in return. My hands wander from her waist down to her ass, which I firmly squeeze. Yes, it is indeed a fabulous ass!

"You have a great ass," I state.

"I know."

I grab her ass and lift her up. She wraps her legs around me. My dipping her makes her giggle. Meanwhile, she is pressing her crotch very tightly against my body, rubbing it up and down. I put her down. She grabs my ass with one hand and moans. I grab her pussy. She moans some more. Then her other hand joins in. She is kneading my ass with both hands. It is time to drag her off.

My first idea is to drag her into one of those booths next to Panoramabar or possibly even straight into the unisex toilet. This triggers sweet memories: not too long ago I met a chick at Berghain who was so horny that I had my dick in her within around ten minutes of meeting her. I railed her hard and then blew a load all over her face. It was awesome. Now that the night is not so young anymore, I decide to play it a bit safer. First, I take her to the sofas right next to Panoramabar. We sit down. I pull her into my lap, which causes her to put one arm around my neck and run her fingertips over my cheek, neck, and chest. I go in for the kiss.

"No, I can't do that," she protests.

"Of course you can!"

I go for the kiss again.

"No, seriously."

I think she is down to fuck. Her nipples are really stiff. I squeeze them through her thin dress. Then I slide one hand in, tickle that magnificent nipple with the tip of my index finger, and finally squeeze one of her fabulous breasts. She is moaning and tries to find my cock. As soon as she locates it she rubs it through my pants. I'm getting pretty hard.

"Wow, you have a really big cock!", she marvels.

I go for the kiss once more. Yet, she averts her mouth yet again.

"Is this too public for you?"

"Nah, I normally really don't mind kissing in public. I do have a reason. It is something different, not what you would expect, but it would take too long to explain it to you. Besides, I do not think we should be talking much anyway."

Her concerns are probably due to a boyfriend or husband at home. Kissing is cheating, but if she does not kiss a guy it is not cheating. It is probably something along those lines. It is similar to how some women claim they are virgins, yet have taken dozens of cocks down their throat or up their ass. I can live with a no-kiss rule.

Her hand is still on my crotch. Instead of just rubbing it she is now squeezing and tugging it. I take this as a prompt to lead her to the unisex toilets. She follows willingly. When I took a dump earlier tonight I noticed two much fairly spacious stalls. They could be intended for the handicapped. As the regular stalls can feel a bit claustrophobic I head to one of the bigger stalls instead. The first one is in use, but the other one is not occupied. I open the door. She quickly walks in. I follow her.

I lock the door. After turning around, I gently but determinedly push her against the wall, which causes a satisfying thud. We stare into each other's eyes. I have one hand in her slutty dress and give her big breasts a tight squeeze, which makes her moan loudly. Now I free one of them and suck on it.

"Uuhhh! Aaahh!", she moans.

Meanwhile, I pull my cock out. She awkwardly tries

getting a hold of it, so I take her hand and put it on it. She grabs it tightly and tugs it. While whacking my cock, she is squatting down in front of me with her legs apart to look even more provocative. Before I know it my cock is all the way in her mouth. It seems that I am in for a treat. She grabs my ass with both hands and vigorously thrusts her head back and forth. In order to support her I grab her by the hair at the back of her head and forcefully ram my cock down her throat, over and over. We are getting a nice rhythm going. After a moment she stalls and takes my cock out of her mouth.

"It would be nicer if you had shaved down there."

"You're probably right," I add. She has a point. Trimming my pubic hair is on my to-do list. I just never get around to it. One of my former fuck buddies even shaved me down there from time to time, but that is not how you form a habit. Anyway, back to the story!

"Yeah, I probably am right," she says with a smile. After a brief pause she follows up with, "Whatever. Let's get this party started!"

She first takes my semi-erect dick fully into her mouth, gently sucks on it until it is hard, and seamlessly transitions into deep-throating again. She does not seem to have a gag reflex. I wonder if I am bruising her throat as I'm fucking her mouth, but that does not take away from my enjoyment. Besides, it is not as if she does not like it. I grab her head with both hands and thrust it back and forth vigorously. When my dick is fully in her mouth she makes gargling sounds that are worthy of a porn starlet and when I pull her head back she wraps her lips tightly around the tip of my cock, sometimes followed by darting her tongue out and sliding it all over my tip. She is really fucking great at this.

After a while I pull my dick out of her ravenous mouth, put my hand on her chin and gesture her to get up. I turn her around, slap her firm ass and grab her panties to pull them down. She stops me. Suddenly, she gets all serious.

"No, stop it. We can't have sex, but I'll do anything else for you."

Unfazed, I grab her pussy. She moans, then she grabs my hand with both of her hands.

"Seriously, we can't fuck. Just let me finish this."

I do not think she is kidding. Well, being a gentleman, I will not force myself upon her. Besides, I needed to get into a more comfortable position anyway.

"Okay, sit down on the toilet," I say to her.

"I'd rather not."

"No problem," I say and lean against the wall. (I would not want to sit down on that disgusting toilet either.) I pull her in and suck on her neck, which she reciprocates. Meanwhile, she is gently stroking my cock, keeping it fully erect.

"But don't leave a mark, do you hear me?", she insists.

I lean in to kiss her.

"I don't want to. Um, I actually would like to. It's more that I can't kiss you."

My curiosity gets the better of me, so I have to ask, "Do you really not like to make out, I mean in general?"

"Normally I do."

I shrug and think that my breath surely cannot be that bad. My dick is still in her hand, so if she does not want to make out with me, she does not want to make out with me.

I put my hand on her head and gently push it to gesture that she should go down on me again. In response, she stands up on her toes and nibbles on my earlobe. Now she is licking and biting my neck and shoulder while tugging my balls. Then she squats down and takes my cock in all the way. She pulls it out again, then she slaps it.

"Mmmm," I moan.

"How do you like that?", she inquires.

She follows this up by spitting on my hard cock and rubbing the spit all over the shaft. Now she is back to deep-throating me like a machine. After a while she pulls my dick out but firmly grabs the base of it with one hand.

"You have a great cock, I really have to say that," she blurts out.

"Glad you like it."

"I'd like to play with it some more, but I think it would turn me on even more to start over and make you come really fast."

I grab her head by her hair with one hand. With the other I take my dick out of her mouth and slap her in the face with it.

"Aaahhh!", she moans.

I slap her again with my cock.

"Aaaahhhhhh!", she responds.

She tries getting a hold of my dick and putting it in her mouth. However, I pull her hair back while I slap her with my hard cock once more.

"Aaaah!"

Now that she has her mouth wide open I shove my cock all the way in. With no holds barred she is sucking me really fast and really well. I lean back against the wall. She is tugging my balls with one hand. With the other she is grabbing my ass. Her technique is excellent: she takes it in all the way quickly and takes it out rather slowly, at which point she uses her tongue to stimulate the shaft. Then she plays with the frenulum before doing a very quick swirl of the tongue over the tip of my cock, followed by wrapping her luscious lips tightly around it and sucking hard on it. She really knows how to suck dick! I bet she finished her Bachelor's in Applied Slut Studies with top grades, *cum laude*. My knees are getting weak. Meanwhile, this sexy scholar is speeding up while she is grabbing my ass harder. Within two minutes or so my dick begins to pulsate.

"I'm about to come," I announce.

Her response is a muffled moaning. I am getting closer and closer to the edge.

"Mmmmm," I moan.

As I am blowing my load I have one hand on the back of her head and fixate it so that my dick is in all the way. I'm getting rid of a big load.

"Mmm! This was so good. You're really good," I say.

She is staring at me with her eyes wide open and my dick still in her mouth. I put my hand away from her head so that she can give her jaw some rest.

Just like in a porn movie she now opens her mouth and reveals that some of my cum is still on her tongue. She sticks her tongue out, then she retracts it again. Now she pushes some cum out of her almost closed mouth. A drip of it slowly runs down from her mouth. She swallows, then she sticks her tongue out to get that one last drop as well.

"That was great. I really liked it," she says.

"Let me do something for you, too," I say as I gesture her to get up. I grab her pussy and rub it. She moans at first but quickly takes my hand away. Then I slide one hand into her panties, squeezing her ass. Moments later I have two fingers in her pussy, which I slowly explore. She arches her back, grabs my wrists with both her hands — and gestures me to stop.

"You really don't have to do this."

"I can't help it."

"No, please stop. It's totally fine. I don't need anything else."

"OK."

"I only wanted to do something nice for you and I am glad I could," she adds with a smile.

"It was great. I should probably say thank you."

"No, you really don't. I should thank you because you just gave me some really hot memories."

We hold and caress each other. She kisses my cheeks before making her way up to my earlobes again. I lean against the wall and enjoy this. Afterward I caress her firm breasts and suck on those magnificent nipples one more time before we wrap our arms around each other again.

"Do you think I am pretty?", she suddenly asks me.

"Yes, you are. You're not just pretty. I think you look spectacular."

"That's so sweet of you to say. Thanks!"

"I don't think a woman like you needs that kind of assurance."

"I don't know. I guess it's just nice to get complimented every once in a while, especially if it's from someone like you."

She has a perfect body, to be quite frank. In order to get more out of this interaction I play with her boobs again.

"I really like your tits," I state.

Hearing this makes her proud. She gives me a huge smile.

"What's your name, by the way?", she asks.

"I'm Aaron."

"Nice meeting you, Aaron. I'm ... ."

Of course I am not going to mention her name, even if it is just her first name. She wraps her arms around me some more and squeezes me tightly.

"I really like your smell, Aaron," she says.

"Thanks."

After a long pause she looks at me.

"This was really fun, but I should probably go find my friends. Is it alright with you if we part ways?"

We leave the spacious toilet for the handicapped and head to the sinks. We wash our hands.

"How does my face look? Do I need to fix my make-up?", she asks.

Berghain does not have any mirrors and the toilets are not lit well enough to make pocket mirrors particularly useful.

"You look fine. Nobody will suspect anything."

"Good."

"Okay, Aaron, time to say goodbye. It was really great meeting you."

"Sure was. How about you give me your number so that we can keep in touch?"

"No, I don't think I can do that."

"Sure. No problem at all."

"Great meeting you. I really mean it!"

"Have fun, sexy!", I say as I hug her. She steps back and smiles. I raise my hand to salute her. Then I turn away but immediately turn around and hurriedly walk after her.

"Wait, can you now tell me why you didn't want to kiss me?"

She laughs.

"Yeah, sure, why not? My husband is a bit of a bore and he only wants to sit at home and relax on the weekend when I would like to go out and party. I felt unhappy sitting at home but after some pleading he agreed to let me go out on my own."

She can barely contain her laughter.

Then she continues, "And you know what, I told him that he does not need to be afraid that I would cheat or anything. I just told him that I will not kiss any guy and that he can trust me on that."

She laughs. I have to laugh as well. (I pity that guy.) She hugs me again.

"Mmm! That smell of yours, Aaron!"

She sniffs my neck and hair, then licks my neck and sucks on it for a moment.

"Okay, this was really fun. But now I have to go," she says.

"Bye. Have fun!"

"I occasionally come to Berghain. Maybe we'll bump into each other again," she adds and winks.

This is it. She walks off. I watch her silhouette disappear in the depths of Berghain.

I take a seat at the sofas outside the unisex toilets and gather my thoughts. As I check my phone I notice that it is only 4:30 a.m. and thus a bit too early to go home. I do not feel like it yet.

How do you feel right after sex? You probably feel re-laxed. If your chick was still around you would cud-dle, do some pillow talk or fall asleep. If she was just a pump-and-dump you might just kick her out but that is another point. Instead, the point is that right after busting a nut I am even more laid-back as I am anyway. Also, after busting a nut in the club I do not really give a fuck anymore and just do what I feel like.

I head back to Panoramabar, where I spot a cute Asian girl, probably Japanese. She is on her own and seems half asleep. I sit down right next to her and immedi-ately put my arm around her waist.

"Come on, this is no time to fall asleep yet," I say.

She smiles.

"Yeah, I know. I'm just taking a break from dancing."

I look her in the eyes. We hold strong eye contact. While holding eye contact I take her drink and pre-tend to take a sip. I do not drink alcohol but she does not know that. She seems to get visibly nervous. The more appropriate term is "aroused." I hand the drink back to her, but she fidgets and spills some over her low-cut top as well as her boobs.

"Now I'm all wet!", she protests with a sassy smile.

She pulls a handkerchief out of her handbag.

"Let me help you out," I say as I take the handkerchief out of her hand.

I slide one hand into her bra to push that nice round breast up and wipe off the alcohol. Then I do the same with the other breast. Well, it is not wet, so I only push it up and squeeze it a bit. "You're so manly," she says while blushing. I'm totally calm and tranquil beyond belief. I could not care less about her reaction, but I sure like touching her boobs.

"Wait," she says.

I lean back expectantly, still having one arm around her waist. She takes her top off. Now I notice that she is wearing two thin tops in a layered manner. The second one comes off as well. Moments later, she is cuddling up to me in her bra. This might sound absurd to you, but you should know that Berghain is a pretty edgy place. You bump into women who dance in tube tops, panties, and heels or knee-high boots. Women dancing in elaborate lingerie and high heels is also not at all uncommon in this place. A few times I have seen women dancing almost naked, with the only piece of clothing being sexy panties.

Her spilling her own drink over herself could well just have been a pretense to join in the fun and show off her great breasts. On those petite Asian girls even a pair of small fake tits looks spectacular. She is clinging onto my arm with both hands. Hesitantly she traces my pectorals.

"You're really manly," she coos.

"Thank you. It's only fitting that you're so feminine, I guess."

She giggles.

I do not consider myself looking particularly manly for Western standards. Compared to the buff faggots on steroids at Berghain I look almost emaciated. Yet, to those slim Asian girls I appear to be hyper-masculine.

"Are you here with some friends?", she asks.

"Nah, I'm out on my own."

"You're so mysterious."

After further giggling she adds, "I'm here with some friends."

Speak of the devil! As she says that, a bunch of Asian guys and girls stand in front of us.

"Here they are!", she shouts.

"Let me introduce you to them," she says.

She gets up. I get up. I hear a bunch of names I absolutely cannot remember or even understand. I thought it is common for Asians to pick an additional English first name to make communication abroad a bit easier.

Well, they either did not or I cannot properly under-stand them. They want to take my girl with them. She gives me a huge smile and extends both hands, gestur-ing me to grab them. I take them and pull her in.

"You're really cute, but I'm getting a bit tired. I don't think I can join your friends," I say.

She pouts.

"For how long are you in Berlin for? Maybe we can hang out next week," I say.

"Yeah, totally. Please take my number!"

We exchange numbers and when her friends are not looking she presses her lips against mine and shoves her tiny tongue into my mouth. Moments later I am watching her lovely little ass disappear in the crowd. Well, that is the downside if you bust a nut in the club. Afterward you may as well go home because you are likely not motivated enough to follow through with some other chick you could bang. I now feel way too tranquil and way too much at ease to really care about getting laid, so I let her go.

I sit down again and doze off for a bit, which is quite an achievement in a loud club. I wake up when someone tries talking to me. I look up. It is some chubby chick with tattoos all over her. I cannot even make out what she says, so I just get up and walk off while she is in mid-sentence. I shudder and head to the exit. I think it is time to leave this place. Making my way slowly through the dance floor, some chick bumps into me sideways and grabs my ass. I turn around. Oh, it is that cock-tease I had met earlier. She seems happy to see me.

"Glad to meet you again, but I have to go to the toilet now," she says.

I understand this to be an invitation, so I take her hand and lead her there. We are in the unisex bathroom. I check the stalls and find an empty one. I wanted to head home, but now that she is making it that easy I may as well see how this will play out. I open the door of one of the stalls and usher her in. I lock the door, turn around and gently push her against the wall. We make out. She is rubbing her pussy up and down my thigh while moaning. I pull her hair and continue with licking and biting her neck.

"Keep going, but I have to tell you that I am a lot of drama," she says.

I really do not like to hear anything like that as it raises a bright red flag. She probably thinks this makes her more attractive. We make out some more. I grab her pussy and rub it.

"Uuhhh," she moans.

Then she snaps out of that, gently pushes me away and says, "Really, it's super-hot that we're now in here, but

I really have to pee now."

"Sure. Go on and pee then."

She laughs, "Yeah, but not with you in here."

I wait outside. She locks the door. A few minutes later she unlocks the door. I open it and walk in. She stands there, giving me this lustful look, and bites her lips. I lock the door again, push her against the wall once more and continue where we had left off. This time I slide my hand into her pants and my middle finger into her wet pussy.

"Aaahhh," she moans.

I pull my cock out and put her hand on it. I am not sure if I am even able to get properly hard, let alone come, considering that I have blown a load quite recently and feel a bit sleepy.

"Give me that cock," she begs.

I gesture her to sit down. The toilet seat does not look any better than the others I have seen tonight. In fact, it looks even worse. Yet, she sits down right away. She grabs my dick and balls with one hand and tugs all of it a bit too aggressively.

"I don't think you know what you're getting into. Do you think you can handle me?", she says.

"We'll see."

"Really, I'm a total mess and very difficult to deal with. No man could handle me yet."

I grab her head and pull her hair.

"Ouch," she says. At the same time she lets go of my cock, so I take it and put it in her mouth. She is sucking on it.

"Mmm," she keeps saying. I slowly get hard, but it is taking me some time.

"Come on, show me how big you can get," she says while looking deep into my eyes.

She keeps sucking me.

"Ouch," I say.

"Sorry, it won't happen again!"

I really do not like feeling teeth on my cock. I lose the erection I had built up so far, so she has to start over. Her rhythm is a bit off. You would expect that the sexually most aggressive women are the best lays and the best cocksuckers, but that is not necessarily the case.

"Watch it," I say as I feel her teeth again.

I hear her mumble, "Sorry."

She keeps sucking my dick. Now the problem is that she is extra careful, so her blowjob just turned into a real slog. I do not think I want to bother much with her, but I let her suck it some more before I take my dick out of her mouth.

"That was good, but I'm getting quite tired. I think I need a break."

"Yeah. But don't tell me you're upset with me. Are you upset?"

"What? No, I'm not. Come on, let's head to the bar."

We fix our clothes and then walk out. The dance floor next to Panoramabar is still packed, so I head right into the crowd and quickly let go of her hand. After, er, accidentally losing her I quickly leave the dance floor and head downstairs. I know she cannot catch up with me because it will take her a lot longer to make her way through the crowd on the dance floor.

The dance floor downstairs is quite busy too. I like the track the DJ put on, so I dance my way through it. As I do so someone grabs my arm. I turn around. It is a girl I pulled a few weeks ago and met up with two or three times since then.

"Aaron, Aaron!", she shouts and jumps up, wrapping her legs around me.

"Hey, great to see you!"

"Do you want to come home with me?"

"I'd love to, but I'm really tired. Not tonight."

She looks disappointed.

"You've got my number. Call me!", she says.

We make out. Then I put her down and walk towards the stairs to the ground floor on my own. That girl is way too high-energy for my taste. I am glad I got off so easily.

As I am walking down the stairs to the exit two tall and very attractive women are making their way up the stairs. I gently run my fingers down the exposed and toned arm of one of them, which she answers with a seductive smile. Some guy walking behind her is not taking this well. He shouts what I presume to be expletives in a foreign language at me and pushes me. I take multiple steps at once a few times before I manage to get a hold of the handrail. I laugh and keep walking. Then I realize that this could have ended quite badly. He could easily have pushed me down the stairs, but to do so forcefully he probably lacked the required strength. With this spike of adrenaline I am leaving the club.

The sun has started to rise already. It is pleasantly warm and the wind gently blows through my hair. It is a perfect morning. Quite frankly, it is a lot nicer without some woman from the club in tow.

Frying Rice

It is Monday and I am back at work, doing a low-paid internship "for the experience." One of my many female colleagues has a nervous breakdown in the office and starts crying uncontrollably, which makes five of the other hens gather around her to comfort her. They get absolutely nothing done for the entire day. Oh, the joys of working in a female-dominated industry! (I have to get out of this.) They took over a meeting room. Later on I see them drinking red wine in the office and eating chocolate, probably put on someone's expense account. Our female boss seems to be fine with them using their work time to eat and drink and comfort each other.

I learned what the issue with my female colleague was. Her now ex-boyfriend told her to pack her things and move out of his apartment. He found out that she has been cheating on him. I did not know that she had a boyfriend. In fact, she aggressively hit on me during my first week in the office. She lives in a really nice part of Berlin-Mitte, in easy walking distance to the office, which I learned about because we once happened to leave work at the same time. She straight-out invited me back to her place to "enjoy a cup of tea together." I found it very uncomfortable when she rubbed her tits against me during lunch earlier that day as it happened in front of a few of my colleagues. She wanted to bang, but banging a colleague is more trouble than it is worth. Imagine her boyfriend had broken up with her because I banged her — I would probably get kicked out right away, with a false sexual harassment or rape accusation thrown at me on top, just so that she can feel better.

After I finish today's work in three hours — roughly what my chatty colleagues routinely take an entire day for — I am tempted to pull a book out of my backpack and read. After all, the women in the office have agreed that no work shall get done today by them. Then I remembered that I have had a pretty good weekend, as you have read in the previous story. I got the phone number of two girls, the Asian one I met at the end of the night and the girl with the skull print on her top, which I met before the night had really started. SKULL deserves her own chapter; flip ahead to the next story if you are impatient. Otherwise, read on to learn about my follow up with that skinny Asian girl with the fantastic fake boobs!

I text her and ask her how she is doing.

"Glad you're alive ;)," she writes back almost immediately, followed by, "I'm leaving tonight. Wanna bang? xxx".

Is she for real? Then I do a double take and notice that she has written "hang", not "bang." In any case, she seems forward. This should be an easy lay even if it probably will not be quite as easy as I would like it to be.

We text back and forth a little bit. A few minutes later I have her room number. She is staying at Park Inn at Alexanderplatz, which is a pretty decent hotel. Four stars, I think. I cannot leave work before 6 p.m., then I am on my way and get a quick bite to eat before taking the underground to Alexanderplatz. At around 6:30 p.m. I knock on her door.

"Open Sesame!," I say.

I hear someone rush to the door.

"Wait, wait!"

The door opens. She stands in front of me in a sexy silk morning robe, presumably not wearing anything underneath. I can see her stiff nipples through the fabric. She jumps up, wraps her legs around my waist and throws her arms around me while saying, "Hi!" I walk into her room with her hanging onto me and close the door behind me. She grabs my head with one hand

and my ass with the other. I remembered her to be a bit taller. She probably wore heels at the club. Now she is standing in front of me. She may not even be five feet tall. She could be 4 ft. 10 in., and thus more petite than the most petite woman I have ever fucked.

"Glad you could come," she says. She leans in. Her tiny tongue darts into my mouth. We make out. I am enjoying this quite a bit, but if she is in that much of a hurry I may as well accelerate the interaction. I walk to the bed and throw her onto it. She sits up, using her elbows as support.

"Come on, undress!", she commands me.

"We don't have any time to waste, don't we?"

"I really don't. I'd love to spend more time with you but my cab to the airport will arrive in less than three hours. What's up with those boring clothes, by the way? That's not how I remember you."

"Work."

"Oh, right."

"Wanna help me out?"

She crawls toward me, then gets on her knees. She unbuttons my shirt, down from the collar, kissing the skin she is exposing. My shirt is on the floor.

"Go on!", I command her.

She unbuckles my belt and pulls it out forcefully, flinging it across the room. She is kissing my abs while she unbuttons my pants. Her tiny hands are now in my briefs. She pulls my dick out, which is getting hard. In her tiny hands it looks gigantic already.

"Wow, you're pretty big," she says.

"Give it a bit more time and you'll be in for a surprise."

She tugs my dick with both hands, which feels unusual. Her fingers are so petite that the sensation is qualitatively different from a when a Western woman with bigger hands does it. I put one hand on her head. With the other I squeeze one of her firm and perky tits. I push her head toward my dick. She takes it into her mouth. There is no resistance whatsoever. Once more, her smallness pays unexpected dividends as the sensation of the tip of her tongue working on the frenulum and tracing the rim of the head of my dick is quite different from what I am used to. She is a precision worker.

Now she tries taking my half-erect dick fully into her mouth. A tear runs down her face as she is shoving it all in. Her lips are wrapped tightly around it and she is moving her head back and forth. All of this feels a bit awkward.

"Come, open your mouth wide," I tell her.

She does so. I grab her head and push it up and down,

skull-fucking her. She is gasping for air. Judging by her loud moans she is clearly enjoying it. After a while I push her head down and my dick all the way in.

"Use your tongue!", I command her.

With my dick down her throat she is sliding her tiny tongue across the shaft of my cock, at least the little she can cover. My cock is getting bigger and bigger. She chokes and has a panicked look on her face. It seems she cannot open her mouth any wider. When my dick is fully erect it touches her teeth. She pulls my dick out of her mouth, panting.

"Holy fuck! Your dick is too big for my mouth. I felt I was about to suffocate."

She is still panting.

"I think there are worse ways to die," I say with a smirk on my face.

"This is not funny," she says while slapping my chest. Then she laughs because it was funny.

She is slowly recovering. I get out of my clothes and hop on her bed. We cuddle for a while and make out. After she has calmed down she caresses my dick with her fingertips.

"I've never seen a cock as big as yours. Not even close."

I am big, but I am not that big.

"Come on now, you must have met other guys who were at least close."

"No, not really. In high school the guys thought I was a nerd and didn't really want me and at my uni there are a lot more women than men, so it's kind of tough to find a guy, even for a one-night stand."

"Bullshit."

"No, really. I'm not a virgin or anything, but we have girls who are, like, really aggressive when going after guys. I don't feel so comfortable doing that so I have not had so many guys yet. I've been with a few, but not with as many as I'd like."

I nod to show sympathy for her plight. She seems to get a bit agitated.

"I mean, it's as if guys don't even see me. I mean, literally. I'm, like, wearing high heels and I still disappear in the crowd. I'm totally invisible. You have no idea what this is like."

Of course I don't, but I nod anyway.

"By the way, when I say men, I mean tall Western men. There are a lot of Chinese and Indian guys at uni but, you know, I really like tall white guys and I'm sure if I wasn't so short I'd do a lot better."

I bend forward, grab one of her round breasts and suck on it. She moans. I come up for air again.

"How come your English is so good, by the way?", I ask.

"My dad's been working all around the world. I had to change school every few years. It's cool because I now know people all over the world."

"Interesting. Is your dad paying for your hotel?"

"Of course," she says with a smile. Daddy's little girl does not need to be exposed to the discomfort of hostels and cheap hotels.

"What are you in Berlin for anyway?", I ask while I am squeezing her ass and she is stroking my dick.

"I'm on a sandwich year at uni. I've just taken a few days off to travel."

"What's a sandwich year?"

"Oh! We take one year off in our four years to work in industry before going back for our final year."

"UK?"

"Yep."

She is at a pretty decent university, pursuing a technical degree. The Asian guys she could get she does not want and the few Western guys she fancies have too many women to choose from who literally throw themselves at them. I think her issue is that she is only aiming for the best the male sex has to offer. Then again, looking at her, I cannot blame her.

"How about you try sucking my dick again?"

My dick has gotten rock-hard in her hands. She opens her mouth wide and wraps her lips around the tip of my cock, sucking on it.

"Go on, take it in deeper!"

Her hands are on the base of my shaft. Her mouth is wide open. She tries getting it all in.

"No, sorry, I really can't," she says, before proceeding to slide her parted lips over my shaft and licking the tip of my cock.

I put one finger in her tight pussy and massage her G-spot. She is moaning while caressing my dick with her lips. She is very wet. I reach for my pants and pull my condoms out. I brought three.

"Here, put this on my dick!", I tell her while I keep fingering her.

She firmly grabs the base of my dick with her left hand. With the right hand she rolls the condom down. From the looks of it she could use a bit more practice.

"I'm kind of scared of your dick because it's so big," she says.

"It'll be fine. Sit down on it!"

I am on my back. She is sitting on me. Now she grabs my dick with one hand, while she supports herself with the other. She is slowly sitting down on my dick, trying to get it into her pussy. We are stuck. I cannot get the tip of my cock in.

"Just try again," I say.

She has a worried look on her face. After a moment I recoil and lose my boner. She tried getting my dick in but her pussy was so tight that the tip of my dick just did not fit. When sitting down on it, using her weight, I sensed a pinching sensation in the tip of my cock, which put a quick end to that attempt. We are back to square one.

My cock looks sad in its flaccid state, sitting in a condom it seems to be too small for.

"I'm sorry, I'm so sorry! Please don't be upset with me!", she pleads.

I stroke her back.

"No big deal. We'll just try again."

After a while I lay her down on her back. I do not want to go down on her, so my fingers have to do. My plan is to warm her up really well and then try again to fuck her. I put one finger in. She is wet enough already. I can tell that with a larger pussy there would have been no issue at all. I put two fingers in. Man, if I had predicted to spend the evening with her I would have packed a bottle of lube in the morning.

"Mmm! Oooohhh!", she moans.

I start working my magic and work on her with two fingers for a few minutes. Now three fingers are in her pussy. At first they barely fit in, but eventually they have enough space. She is writhing and arching her back. Let us see if I can make her come this way! I keep going.

"Aaaaahhh! Aaaahhhhh! Aaaaaa!"

Yup, she is coming alright. She is one of the quickest I have ever met.

Seeing this super-sexy body being shaken by orgasmic shockwaves is turning me on quite a bit. She has not gotten a lot wetter but I have stretched her pussy out a bit, which should help. I put another condom on. She is on her back. I am about to mount her. She puts both hands on my midriff, presumably so that she can easily indicate when I am in too deep. Well, for that to happen, I first have to get in. I lift up one of her legs. Now I try sliding my cock in. She is still amazingly tight, too tight even. I spit into my hands twice, then rub the spit over my cock. I try again. After one vigorous push I am finally in. The toughest part was getting the tip of my cock in there and now that that is done I can start fucking her — or so I think.

As I am getting my dick in she lets out a loud moan. I pull my pelvis back and slowly push my cock all the way in afterward. Her moans quickly turn into a loud, "Ouch."

"What's the matter?", I ask.

"Don't worry, keep going, but don't go in too deep, please!"

I am carefully pounding her. After a good two minutes, I do another hard thrust.

"Ouuaaaaahhh!", she moans.

I stop. Then I pound her slowly, with my dick only going in about halfway. I do this for a few minutes. I would love to smash her pussy hard, but I do not want to hurt this fragile creature.

"Fuck me hard, please!", she begs.

"Finally," I think.

I am hammering away. From what I can tell it is still a bit painful for her when I go in all the way, but she seems to really enjoy it. I am pounding her rhythmically. She is so into it that I see the white of her eyes. For a moment I worry that I am pounding her unconscious. I cannot say that I am not enjoying myself. It is clear that she is getting a lot more enjoyment out of it than I. She is having the time of her life, getting impaled by my big cock.

I have pounded her enough now and I want to come, so I pull out and the condom off. She quickly jumps up, grabs my cock and strokes it while opening her mouth and sticking her tongue out. Then she stops.

"Do you have any condoms left?", she asks.

"I got one left."

"Then you'll fuck me again!"

She puts my dick away, disappears into the bathroom and comes back with some wet tissues.

"I don't like the taste of condoms," she says while cleaning my cock. She licks the shaft afterward, then stops.

"I still taste it. Let's take a shower!"

She grabs my dick and leads me into the shower that way, soaps up my entire body, and properly cleans it. Her tiny hands feel really great. Eventually she puts my flaccid dick in her mouth while I am still in the shower. As soon as I am getting harder she takes it out of her mouth and licks the shaft.

We dry each other. Then we go for another round.

"Can you do me doggy?", she asks.

"I don't think that's such a good idea."

"Pleeeassseeee!"

"Are you sure you can take it?"

"Pretty pleeease!"

She gets down on her knees and puts her ass in the air. I finger her first; once I have stretched her out enough with three fingers I put my last condom on and slide my dick in, which is just as difficult as before. Okay, here we go again! When I am pounding her deep she screams. Her head is on the pillow sideways, so I can see the pain on her face.

"I'm sorry, I can't take it when you go in all the way," she whimpers.

I fuck her shallowly for a while, but that is not nearly as much fun, neither for me nor her. I pull out and flip her over on her back and mount her. Then I put my dick in and hammer away. There is the same strangely satisfying mixture of an expressions of pain and lust on her face. She is getting a lot more into it. First she only puts her hands on my ribcage. Then her hands are on my back, caressing it. Moments later she is trying to grab the flesh.

We fuck in a great rhythm. My hard deep thrusts work in unison with her pushing back hard. I'm in a trance-like state. Then she scratches me!

"Ouch!", I scream.

"Don't be such a pussy!", she says.

In response I grab one of her firm ass cheeks hard. I keep pounding her. She now scratches my back whenever I go in deep. Unexpectedly, I quickly take a liking to the pain. Judging from looking at her face she feels more pain (and lust) than me, though.

I am getting close to an orgasm, so I pull out and stroke myself. She gets up and on her knees, looking at my dick expectantly while biting her lip. Then I blow a load all over her face, which makes her look at me in a really horny expression. She slowly licks my dick afterward, while my cum is running down her face.

I collapse on the bed. She rests her cum-covered face on my chest and coos, "That was totally mind-blowing. Phew!"

I am still panting.

"Don't get this the wrong way, but I'm kind of glad it's over," she adds.

"What do you mean?"

"Well, I really had no idea for how much longer I could take it. A few times I was afraid I'd pass out. I'm not kidding."

I smile.

We both fall asleep.

❦

The alarm rings.

"Shit, shit, shit!", she says.

I slowly open my eyes and see her panicking, with my dried cum on her face. I chuckle.

"Quick, get up! My cab will arrive in 15 minutes!"

"I think you should take a shower," I say to her.

"Shit!"

"Come with me, we'll do it together!"

We take a quick shower and dry each other.

I get dressed while she uses a hairbrush to get some dry cum out of her hair.

"I'm so glad that I have packed already."

She collects her things, still naked. Then she quickly dresses.

"I don't need a lot of makeup, so I'll apply that in the cab. What about you? Do you have everything?"

"Yup."

She slips into a pair of jeans and a pink sweater before putting on sneakers.

"I'd be so fucked if I had to wear heels and a dress right now," she comments.

We take the elevator down to the lobby. She checks out.

"Do you mind waiting with me for the cab?"

"Sure, no problem."

Just about two minutes later, her cab rolls up. She looks at me, puts her hands on my shoulders and stands on her toes. I bend down. She kisses me on my lips.

"Thank you. That was great!", she says.

"Sure was."

I bend forward to kiss her properly. I once again feel her tiny tongue darting into my mouth. We make out briefly.

"You have a flight to catch."

"I know."

"Take care!"

"Take care, and good luck!"

I turn around to leave.

"Wait!"

"Yes?"

She gets up on her toes and whispers in my ears, "I enjoyed being your obedient slut."

The Lingerie Model

Two stories ago I told you about that amazingly hot woman I called SKULL. That was last Saturday. Now it is Monday and I have not gotten laid in two days, so I call her during a break at work. She picks up the phone immediately.

"Oh my god, Aaron! I'm so glad you're calling," she squeaks.

I could tell that she has a big smile on her face. It feels like a done deal already.

"I'm surprised you remember my name," I jest.

"I bet you don't remember putting it in my phone. I later added 'Berghain maniac' to it."

"Am I supposed to feel flattered by it?"

"I don't know," she says and giggles.

"Listen, how about we hang out some time this week, maybe Wednesday?", I suggest.

"That would be great! What do you want to do?"

"We'll see. Can you meet me at 6:30 p.m. at Alexanderplatz, under the World Time ... ?"

"The World Time Clock is such a cliche. All the singles meet there," she responds and laughs.

"I didn't know that. Anyway, we can just grab two girls from there and have an orgy. What do you say?"

She laughs, "I hope I'll be enough for you."

"Alright. See you then!"

"Wait!," she says with a serious tone.

"Yes?"

"Um, do you do this a lot, I mean, picking up girls in clubs, having orgies and whatnot?"

Orgies? I must have made quite an impression on her if she believes that I can just grab a bunch of random chicks, take them home, and have an orgy.

"I wish. Anyway, see you!"

"Yeah, see you soon!"

It is Wednesday. Work was a drag but now I am on the way to Alexanderplatz. After a dull day spent in the office, banging a hot girl is just what I need.

I am a few minutes late and so is she, it seems. As I cross the street to walk toward the World Time Clock someone shrieks and shouts my name. I turn around. It is probably her. I remember her looking differently. In the club she had her hair open, wore a tube top that accentuated her breasts, and had plenty of make-up on her face. Her bright red lipstick also sent all the right signals. Now, in broad daylight and dressed like a regular girl she does not draw nearly as much attention.

She greets me with an enthusiastic shriek and throws her arms around me. We hug tightly. Immediately afterward she puts her hand on my biceps, which I flex in response.

"Just like I remember you," she coos.

I smile.

"So, where are you going to take me, big boy?"

"I'll look for an alley."

She laughs, "That's not what I meant."

I shrug, take her hand and lead her off.

"You're not serious, are you? I can't believe this," she says and giggles.

After a few steps she brushes some real or imaginary lint off my jacket, which is a great sign. Moments later I stop and turn toward her. She looks me in the eyes, like a deer in headlights. I lift her chin up with my index and middle fingers before I slowly kiss her. After a while she comes up for air.

"Right, we haven't done this yet."

Before I can say anything in response she tongues me down. It's on like Donkey Kong! My first idea was to take her to a bar, but the weather is too pleasant to sit inside. Instead, we walk toward the town hall of Berlin, Rotes Rathaus. While enjoying the evening sun we chit-chat. I am on autopilot. Besides, when I talk with random women I just say whatever I feel like anyway.

"You know, you remind me somewhat of my former French teacher, except you are way hotter," I say.

"Is this a compliment?"

"Most certainly. I kind of had a crush on her. I spent more time jerking off, thinking of her, than doing my homework."

She giggles. We make deep eye contact while I play with her hair. After a long and sexy smile she starts blabbing in French, probably something naughty. I do not understand a single word because the pathetically little French I know is more than rusty.

"My only recollection of French is Emmanuelle's ass, so cut it out," I say with a smirk.

More French is coming out of her mouth.

"Alright, then," I say as I cover her mouth with one hand.

"Mmm. Mmmm."

I put my hand away. She giggles and I can see that she is blushing a little bit. This tells me that she responds very well to being dominated.

We stand in front of a bench. I sit down. She pretends that she is about to sit down in my lap, but then she gets up again, puts her hands on my shoulder and kisses me once more.

"On a first date I better behave and sit down next to you instead."

She sits down next to me. The first thing she does is put both hands on my thigh. I am getting hard. I return that favor by putting one hand on her thigh, close to her crotch. Every once in a while I accidentally brush across her breasts.

As we blab on we learn that we have some biographical similarities as we both grew up in a relatively sheltered environment. That is not too surprising, considering that Berlin is full of people who want to leave their past behind and reinvent themselves. Unfortunately, instead of attempting to reinvent themselves most just take their provincial mindset with them.

The conversation steers toward sex, probably because I put her hand on my crotch. She notices my erection, so she eagerly massages my cock through the fabric of my pants.

"Don't make me blow a load," I say.

"Isn't that what you want?"

"Sure, but not here."

She smiles mischievously.

"Have you ever, um, done anything at Berghain beyond dancing?", she inquires.

"Sure."

That seems to be all the information she wants to know, judging by her tight grip on my cock. Since we are enjoying such a highly sexual vibe, it is about time we move this interaction elsewhere.

"Do you live alone?", I ask her.

"I do," she says with a subsequent giggle, before adding, "But I don't bring guys home on the first date."

"That's alright. I only want to cuddle anyway," I say. This is of course bullshit, but it is the kind of bullshit girls use when they want to have sex with you but do not want to be too explicit. She knows what's up and giggles some more.

"I have to know if I really like someone before doing anything sexual, you know?"

Judging by the fact that she is squeezing my cock she seems to really like me. My boner is quite discomforting, so I pull my dick out and hide it under my shirt.

She immediately grabs it again. I can tell that she is hugely turned on, not just because she gets to play with my dick for real but also because we are in broad daylight with people walking past in front and behind us.

She finds a creative way to sexually stimulate me without raising any suspicions. I have more than a hunch that she is quite experienced. She positions my dick sideways and removes her hand from under my shirt. Now her hand is on my shirt, pressing down on the shaft of my dick. Her thumb is on top of the tip of my cock, which she gently rubs in a circular motion. In between she administers the occasional proper stroke. Apparently she is getting too turned on by me rubbing her crotch.

This goes on for a while. Then she takes her hand away from my cock. I give her some respite before I nonchalantly take her hand and put it on my cock again. She gives me this horny look and then says, "You give off a very slight smile when you do this. It's as if you are saying that it's just a game and that it's cool if I play along." That is a tad too philosophical for my taste, so I just lean back and enjoy her rubbing my hard cock through my shirt. I have not been aware of that particular kind of smile.

Getting your genitals rubbed is all well and good, but consenting adults probably want more than that. It struck me that the main building of Humboldt University is within walking distance. It is a pretty run-down place, befitting the ultra-leftwing orientation of many of its students. There are parts of the building that smell rotten, which includes, to my astonishment, a smaller lecture hall that is occasionally used for public lectures. It is as if the administration does not care about public perception at all.

"Have you seen the yard of Humboldt University? It's a beautiful place," I say.

That would be true if it were not swarming with smelly left-wing students with dreadlocks. Then again, at this hour the university is probably empty.

"No, but I bet you are now going to take me there!"

"Indeed I will."

It took us just a few minutes to get there. There was a demonstration earlier today, which was partly organized by Humboldt students. Accordingly, the surrounding area of the university is a complete mess, the yard in particular. The main building of the university has been in disarray probably ever since the times of the former German Democratic Republic. At the very least its façade should be properly cleaned, but with the leftists in power in Berlin this is not going to happen anytime soon. The yard looks particularly unappealing, with trash strewn all over the grass. It is a far cry from the cozy and romantic recluse it can be at dusk that I remembered. Those commie revolutionaries now expect a bunch of supposedly privileged white men to clean up after them.

As much as I like to bitch about Germany in general and Berlin in particular I should not be too judgmental, considering that I am enrolled at that university myself. For a little over 200 euros per semester you get access to free or heavily subsidized healthcare and a free ticket for public transport. Socialism is not so bad if you are a leech. You do not even have to take any classes. On that note, when I enrolled I mistook a student for an employee. He then proudly told me that he is about to re-enrol himself and that he has been studying History for forty semesters. Since there are two semesters per year this means that he has been enrolled for twenty years.[4]

As we are walking around the building I share this story and others. I also know a bit about the history of the place and a few anecdotes, which I relay to her. She is lapping it up.

"How can someone so obviously smart and educated like you not have a proper job?", she asks me.

"That's a long story."

---

[4]Regulations have been tightened recently. I think you now have ten years to finish a degree before they kick you out, but of course you can just enroll in another degree program to reset the clock.

We cross the yard and enter the main building. We stand in front of the main staircase, which splits into two stairs. It displays a quotation by Karl Marx in big letters at its bifurcation point, thus defacing the beautiful red marble of the foyer. It roughly translates to, "The philosophers have only interpreted the world differently. However, it is more important to change it." I read it out loud with audible disdain.

"There is no value in change for its own sake. On the other hand, you could make a good argument that you need stability for prosperity, which is nicely reflected, perhaps surprisingly so, in Schumpeter's idea of creative destruction," which I briefly summarize for her. She marvels and listens. Then she smiles and opens her mouth again.

"Since when do big cocks come with big brains?"

I slap her ass playfully in response.

"Don't mock me for imparting my wisdom on you."

"I'm not. I'm impressed."

I gently push her against one of the pillars in the foyer. We make out. I grab her pussy and rub it. Her fingers are grazing the bulge in my pants. It is about time I capitalize on her horniness and I am too impatient to head back to my place or hers. So, let us aim for the bathrooms! I have to pee anyway. It would probably alienate her if I dragged her into a bathroom stall and first made her watch me pee. My other option is to enter one of the bathroom stalls on my own, walk out, and drag her inside. This is not smooth either.

I take her hand and tell her that I have to pee. I am heading toward one of the restrooms in the east wing of the building. Those places are not unisex, but I do not have the impression that there is anyone in the building at this time anyway. I open the door and take her with me. Inside, I push her against the wall and tongue her down hard.

"I'll be right back," I say to her as I open the doors to one of the stalls.

"OK. I'll wait right here," she replies, looking at me doe-eyedly.

I take a piss, flush, and head out. Seconds later I grab her, push her against the wall and tongue her down again. Meanwhile, I open the door to the bathroom stall I just exited and guide her inside. She follows willingly. As I lock the door she moans slightly in anticipation. She is already getting very turned on.

I push her against the wall and rub her crotch. While making out with her I unbuckle my belt and pull my pants down. Both her hands are instantly on my cock. The passion is palpable. I think that this is a really cool situation. It is similar to a lot of my club hookups, but it feels nothing like it. I have to say that I quite like skull-fucking a chick to the beat of the music, but that is not going to happen.

Someone opens the door to the bathroom and walks in. It is some dude taking a piss. I do not want to attract undue attention, so I gesture her to be quiet. She gently strokes my dick as we listen to someone wash his hands and heading out. Okay, time to get going again. I pull her top down and free one of her tits. Licking that nipple makes her moan heavily. I expect the chances of someone else walking in to be quite low, so I do not cover her mouth and let her keep moaning.

I gesture her to get up and turn her around. I grab her pants and pull them down. Moments later she has my middle finger in her tight pussy.

"Aaahhhh!", she moans.

Judging from her squirming movements she is enjoying this quite a bit. I turn her around again and put my hands on her shoulders to indicate that she should sit down.

"I'm not going to blow you in here," she says.

I smirk, turn her around, and finger her hard. She is moaning loudly and vigorously pushes her pelvis back, synchronized with the thrusts of my hand. I would say that we are getting along really well. I stop and nonchalantly pull out a condom. I tear open the wrapper and put it on.

"What are you doing? Are you crazy?", she objects.

"Yeah, I am."

She laughs.

"No, seriously, we're not going to fuck in here."

To underscore her statement she pulls the condom off my cock and throws it on the ground with a smile. She sits down on the toilet again, holding my cock between her palms. After looking at my fully erect penis for a while she puts her lips on the tip of my cock and slowly takes it into her mouth. She is sucking it well. To make this more of a team effort I put one hand on the back of her head and guide it toward me when I am thrusting. To my chagrin I am not getting any deep-throat action.

The door to the bathroom opens again. This really is nothing like a club bathroom pull. She gets up and whispers, "Considering that I originally did not want to blow you and that I don't do such things on the first date anyway, this is way too much already." The big smile on her face tells a different story, though. Meanwhile, we listen to another dude taking a piss. He is quick. That filthy pig did not even wash his hands. Now that he is gone I shove her into the wall and kiss her passionately. She still has one hand on my dick. I sit her down again.

She puts my dick in all the way and administers a technically very impressive blowjob. No pun intended, but

I am quite blown away by how she goes from sucking it slowly to increasing the speed very smoothly. A lot of girls suck you at only a constant speed; the more experienced ones know the difference between fast and slow, but only very few go beyond that. I would not be surprised if she has done some whoring on the side because that level of skill normally requires experience with more than a few cocks.

She is getting faster and faster. My cock is starting to throb. She stops. It seems she does not want me to blow a load. Yet, I have been looking forward to doing that, preferably on her face. Gripping my cock, she is looking at me.

"Do you want to come?", she asks me.

I smirk.

"But what about me?"

I gesture to her to get up. With one aggressive motion I pull her pants and panties down simultaneously. She ends up with two fingers in her pussy. I finger her forcefully with my index and middle finger. During this she deeply gazes into my eyes, like in a trance. It is beautiful. She comes quickly and embraces me tightly as she lets out one moan after another. I let her pant for a while. Before I get the chance to take control of the situation again she sits down and gets right back to sucking my dick. It does not take long before my dick starts to throb again. I take my dick out of her mouth and keep whacking it.

"Show me your tongue!", I command her.

Obligingly she opens her mouth and sticks her tongue out. I press the tip of my cock against her tongue and keep jerking it. I am getting close. Yes, there it is! I shoot a nice big load right into her mouth. It would have made for a great video. As soon as I am done blowing my wad she wraps her lips around the tip of my cock and sucks hard on it for a while. Then she rummages in her handbag and pulls out a pack of tissues. After spitting my cum into some tissue paper she throws it into the toilet bowl. This is not the time to explain to her that tissue paper can clog a toilet, so I ignore it. However, she interprets my skeptical look differently.

"I only swallow when I really, really like someone," she explains.

Yup, she probably has sucked a lot of dick in her life. Of course it is nice when some chick swallows your load, but the difference between a chick sucking and spitting it out after coming in her mouth versus her sucking and swallowing it afterward is quite negligible when the alternative is not getting your dick sucked at all. To her, though, it seems that there is a meaningful difference between swallowing or not. I want to chuckle but manage to suppress it. Besides, I could not care less about whether she swallows or not as long as she keeps sucking my cock while I ejaculate in her mouth. She is good at that, too.

We fix our clothes, caress each other for a bit, and then head back out again. While I am washing my hands, my phone vibrates. After drying my hands I check my phone. It was BYTE. I text him that I am busy tonight.

A little later we are on the way to the staircase. We hear some music playing, which leads us to an evening reception. Looking at the crowd, it seems that we will fit in.

"Let's crash it," I say to her.

"Yeah, let's do it!", she says and giggles.

Moments later we are feasting on a succulent buffet, funded by taxpayers' money. She is now completely comfortable in my company and even more once she has gotten a bit to drink. We hang out for another two hours, eating and drinking and sitting and talking. I enjoy my time with her. We have great rapport and she certainly knows how to keep a guy interested. At one point I notice her fingers under my shirt. A little later she scratches me gently.

The more time we spend together, the more confident she gets. However, when she gets up on her toes and bites my neck in an inappropriate situation I know that it is time to leave. One hour later we are back at her place. There, I am taken aback by a column of pictures of sexy legs and torsos.

"What's up with that?", I ask her.

"That? That's me! I've been doing lingerie modeling for a while now."

I take another look and notice the similarity. Minutes later we are in her bedroom. She is on all fours and I am pounding the shit out of her. Afterward, she really, really liked me.

❦

SKULL was an amazing chick — at first. I banged her for about two weeks and enjoyed myself tremendously. Eventually it fell apart, quickly and unexpectedly. This is how it went down: I head to her place on Thursday after work. She opens the door in her morning robe. We make out passionately. Moments later we are in her bed. My cock is in her hands.

"Wait, before we do anything, I want to ask you something," she says.

"Anything you want."

"I would like us to go steady, like, you know, boyfriend and girlfriend."

"So you are trying to squeeze the answer out of me, aren't you?"

She laughs and lets go of my cock.

"No, I'm dead serious. I want you to commit."

"I'm not sure this is the right time."

She looks at me.

"Come here," I say as I try embracing her.

She pushes me back and looks at me like a crazy person. I am getting the chills.

"What's your answer?", she asks.

"I don't like being put on the spot."

I start to feel really uncomfortable. She gets up.

"Okay," she mumbles.

She collects my clothes.

"Wait, I can do that myself," I say.

She throws my clothes at me and shouts, "So you only wanted to fuck me? Is that it? Really, is that it?"

"Chill out!"

"Take your clothes and get the fuck out!"

I am in the hallway, getting dressed. She stands in front of me and is right in my face.

"You're such an asshole. I thought you liked me. Hell, I thought I liked you."

I do not say anything. Instead, I hurriedly get dressed. Then I walk to the door to get my shoes.

"That's right, just walk away. Walk the fuck away you fucking asshole! You fucking piece of shit!"

She seems a bit deranged to me. I want to get the hell out so I grab my shoes and rush down the stairs to the foyer of her apartment building in my socks. I hear the door slam and hope that she will stay inside instead of coming after me. I really do not want to have to deal with her in public. Thankfully, that does not happen. After putting on my shoes I head to the nearest station to get home.

The next day I receive a long and apologetic email from her. She writes that she is sorry that she overreacted, gushes over what a great guy I am, "with your smarts and your regal height," and that we would make a wonderful couple. She justifies her behavior by feeling pressure because she is about to turn 27 soon and "feels" that she needs to settle down.

I will let you in on a sad secret: passionate women are great in the sack. However, the other side of the coin is that passionate women tend to be emotionally unstable. If you fall in love with such a woman, chances that you will get fucked in a very bad way are sky-high. Some women with mental problems play their cards a lot better. That one did not. What is worse, if I did not have other women around to fuck, it is possible that I would have gone back to her because it is quite rare to have a woman who not only looks spectacular but who is also great in bed. I dodged a bullet.

www.ingramcontent.com/pod-product-compliance
Lightning Source LLC
Chambersburg PA
CBHW022357280326
41935CB00007B/218